diminished and rational evidence dismissed, simply because at a certain time or

times I lost contact with the consensus of reality agreed on by my peers, then it is

scarcely possible to expect that my control over my life will ever be less than

severely circumscribed. If my experience is not valued I cannot be whole.

It is currently quite unclear whether those who work in the psychiatric system

place a high priority on maximising an individual's self-control during the process of

breakdown. In this respect I find it significant that no psychiatric professional has

ever advised me on how to cope with a breakdown beyond the blanket

exhortation to keep on taking the drugs. My own experiences suggest that once I

start to lose control again I am expected to admit powerlessness, hand myself over

to the experts and count to fifteen thousand. Such suspicions tend to be

confirmed by the notably frosty reception my own ideas about my treatment

recieve from those who are attempting to process me back to in-patient status.

It is clear to me that it is inconvenient to have to consider the integrity of

the new admission too carefully during absorption into the psychiatric system.

It is clear to me that the systems' needs dominates the individual's needs.

Whatever the intentions behind the system. the reality

AT THE HEART OF A MAD MOVEMENT

This book showcases and celebrates the writings of Peter Campbell, an activist, writer, educator, and a veteran survivor of the mental health system, conveying the variety and vitality of Campbell's accomplishments across the years from 1967 to 2022.

Diagnosed with severe psychosis and with a history of hospitalizations reaching back to 1967, Peter Campbell was an indefatigable critic of orthodox psychiatry and of many aspects of the mental health system. He was a founder and veteran of the groundbreaking psychiatric survivors' movement in 1980s and 1990s Britain. The diverse essays within this book cover topics such as seclusion, spiritual crisis, lived experience of psychosis, ECT and psychiatric drugs, and the survivor movement, together with a number of in-depth interviews, as well as other creative contributions such as dramatic scripts and satirical sketches. Brought together, these diverse creations are an eloquent testimony to the humanity, unflagging commitment and staying power of a hugely significant writer, innovator, commentator, and critic.

Written in Campbell's accessible and witty style, this will be an invaluable resource for practitioners in psychiatry and all disciplines, people with lived experience of psychosis and their relatives and carers, activists, and all concerned with distress and mental wellbeing.

Peter Barham is a psychologist and historian of mental health. He has been working, writing, and engaging critically, in the mental health field for more than 50 years. His work straddles clinical research, psychoanalysis, practical initiative, historical inquiry, mental health activism, and film making. He is a Fellow of the British Psychological Society, and founder of the Hamlet Trust, which pioneered grassroots mental health reform in Eastern Europe.

Peter Beresford OBE is Visiting Professor at the University of East Anglia and Co-Chair of Shaping Our Lives, the national disabled people's and service users' organization and network. He is also Emeritus Professor of Social Policy at Brunel University London and the University of Essex. He was awarded the Honorary Degree of Doctor of Science by Edge Hill University, in 2017. He is a long-term user of mental health services and has a longstanding background of involvement in issues of participation as writer, researcher, activist, and teacher. He has published more than 30 books and many journal articles and book chapters, as well as contributions to mainstream journalism.

Ker Wallwork is an artist and the project archivist for the Peter Campbell Legacy Project, hosted by the Bishopsgate Institute. Previously they worked with members of the Survivors History Group to provide digital access to the archives of the Mental Patients Union and ensure the preservation of a range of survivor and disability related archives.

THE INTERNATIONAL SOCIETY FOR PSYCHOLOGICAL AND SOCIAL APPROACHES TO PSYCHOSIS BOOK SERIES

Series editor: Anna Lavis

Established over 50 years ago, the International Society for Psychological and Social Approaches to Psychosis (ISPS) has members in more than 20 countries. Central to its ethos is that the perspectives of people with lived experience of psychosis, their families and friends, are key to forging more inclusive understandings of, and therapeutic approaches to, psychosis.

Over its history ISPS has pioneered a growing global recognition of the emotional, sociocultural, environmental, and structural contexts that underpin the development of psychosis. It has recognized this as an embodied psychosocial experience that must be understood in relation to a person's life history and circumstances. Evidencing a need for interventions in which listening and talking are key ingredients, this understanding has distinct therapeutic possibilities. To this end, ISPS embraces a wide spectrum of approaches, from psychodynamic, systemic, cognitive, and arts therapies, to need-adapted and dialogical approaches, family and group therapies and residential therapeutic communities.

A further ambition of ISPS is to draw together diverse viewpoints on psychosis, fostering discussion and debate across the biomedical and social sciences, as well as humanities. This goal underpins international and national conferences and the journal *Psychosis*, as well as being key to this book series.

The ISPS book series seeks to capture cutting edge developments in scholarship on psychosis, providing a forum in which authors with different lived and professional experiences can share their work. It showcases a variety of empirical focuses as well as experiential and disciplinary perspectives. The books thereby combine intellectual rigour with accessibility for readers across the ISPS community. We aim for the series to be a resource for mental health professionals, academics, policy makers, and for people whose interest in psychosis stems from personal or family experience.

To support its aim of advancing scholarship in an inclusive and interdisciplinary way, the series benefits from the advice of an editorial board:

For more information about this book series, visit www.routledge.com/The-International-Society-for-Psychological-and-Social-Approaches-to-Psychosis/book-series/SE0734

For more information about ISPS, email isps@isps.org or visit our website, www.isps.org.

For more information about the journal *Psychosis* visit : https://isps.org/publications/isps-journal/

AT THE HEART OF A MAD MOVEMENT

The Life and Work of Peter Campbell,
Psychiatric System Pioneer

*Edited by Peter Barham,
Peter Beresford and Ker Wallwork*

Routledge
Taylor & Francis Group

LONDON AND NEW YORK

Designed cover image: From a drawing by Peter Campbell of Minstead
Lodge, January 1986, copyright the estate of Peter Niall Campbell.

First published 2026
by Routledge
4 Park Square, Milton Park, Abingdon, Oxon OX14 4RN

and by Routledge
605 Third Avenue, New York, NY 10158

Routledge is an imprint of the Taylor & Francis Group, an informa business

British Library Cataloguing-in-Publication Data
A catalogue record for this book is available from the British Library

Library of Congress Cataloging-in-Publication Data
Names: Campbell, Peter, 1949 January 3- author. | Barham, Peter editor |
Beresford, Peter editor | Wallwork, Ker editor
Title: At the heart of a mad movement : the life and work of Peter
Campbell, psychiatric system pioneer / edited by Peter Barham, Peter
Beresford and Ker Wallwork.
Description: Abingdon, Oxon ; New York, NY : Routledge, 2026. | Series:
The international society for psychological and social approaches to
psychosis book series | Collection of writings by Peter Campbell from
1967 to 2022. | Includes bibliographical references and index.
Identifiers: LCCN 2025020526 (print) | LCCN 2025020527 (ebook) |
ISBN 9781041066477 hardback | ISBN 9781041066453 paperback |
ISBN 9781003636434 ebook
Subjects: LCSH: Campbell, Peter, 1949 January 3---Mental health. |
Psychiatric hospital patients--Care--Great Britain. | Mental health
policy--Great Britain. | Psychiatric hospital care--Great Britain. |
Health activism--Great Britain.
Classification: LCC RC464.C27 A25 2026 (print) | LCC RC464.C27 (ebook)
LC record available at https://lccn.loc.gov/2025020526
LC ebook record available at https://lccn.loc.gov/2025020527

ISBN: 978-1-041-06647-7 (hbk)
ISBN: 978-1-041-06645-3 (pbk)
ISBN: 978-1-003-63643-4 (ebk)

DOI: 10.4324/9781003636434

Typeset in Times New Roman
by KnowledgeWorks Global Ltd.

CONTENTS

0.1

LIST OF ILLUSTRATIONS

Photographs of Peter Campbell

1   Photograph of Peter Campbell in the 'Ham & High' newspaper, to accompany article 'Anger breaks through the psychiatric wilderness', 11 September 1987, licence to use the picture by Newsquest.
2   Frank Bangay, Andrew Roberts and Peter Campbell, founding members of the Survivors' History Group, at the Bunhill Quaker Meeting House, 29 August 2008. Photographed by Frank Baron and printed in *The Guardian*, 3 September 2008. Reproduction licence granted by Eyevine Ltd.
3   Peter Campbell performing 'The Mental Marching Band' at Kingsley Hall, Bow, East London, 19 March 2010, photographed by Nat Fonnesu & reproduced with permission.

'Melvin Menz' cartoon series by 'Niall' for the *Survivors Speak Out* newsletter [2.04]

'A danger to yourself!'
'Supervised discharge'
'A constructive mid-field'
'Assertive outreach'.

'Bin Busters' cartoon by 'Niall' (pseudonym of Peter Campbell)

0.2

FOREWORD

'They all smiled
But the drapes were down
Thirteen nutters seen this morning
Even the constitutional niceties
Sometimes wear thin.

She did not smile
Sat next to me
Erect
In black
With Doc Martens boots on.

"We would get on much better, doctor,
If you didn't keep interrupting him".

There was a pause
The shifting of spines

A page in my history
Turning irreversibly
Forwards'
        Crisis Advocate, Peter Campbell

I remember the first time I met Peter, he was enamoured by my middle name (Roxanne) and I was immediately struck by his searing intelligence, gentle demeanour, and a twinkle in his eye which I later found accompanied a brilliant sense of humour.

We shared a lot of laughter at ourselves, the state of psychiatric services and the world at large. Peter was one of the most important influences on me as a young woman and activist. He listened intently – to everyone – that in itself made him stand out to me.

I soon discovered a humble man without edge or ego who lifted others up. He facilitated opportunities for others, always inclusive, putting others forward, and was a nurturing mentor, inviting participation in his workshops, so you could dip your toe into the water, knowing you had a mind guard of steel sitting beside you.

He wanted to know about people, their truths and experiences, and he encouraged everyone to fulfil their potential be it writing, speaking, teaching. Peter was a deep thinker, some of my fondest memories of him were us chewing the fat about mental health politics, activism and survivor led approaches. Peter embodied a style of leadership you rarely see, I can just see his frown at my saying 'leader', but he was a towering leader, laying the foundations for others after him.

When he recited his poetry to a nursing congress, the connection with the audience was palpable. *Brown Linoleum Green Lawns* remains my all-time favourite poetry book. 'Crisis Advocate', a poem he wrote about and for me, is an accurate description of me being Peter's mind guard in a Care Planning Approach (CPA) meeting. He captured that moment eloquently. I was late 20s when I sometimes acted as his mind guard at CPA meetings. It's a natural thing to do with good friends, just as he sometimes accompanied me to A&E.

We did some sessions together, I can't remember where, on our experiences of bipolar (Manic Depression then) for Peter, and psychosis (I was initially diagnosed with schizophrenia & catatonia) for me. I remember walking around with him when he was manic, and because he was tall and long limbed, I'd have to scurry fast to keep up with him! We ended up in a church once and in his mind we had married. We would share a laugh about these moments after, we always shared some humour, or dark humour.

I called Peter once after an especially hard conference because of a professional's abusiveness, and there he was at the station, ready to sit with me over a cuppa and tissues, helping me to learn how to navigate these scenarios. Peter was always the first person to visit friends in hospital. That's the kind of man, friend, and activist Peter was, always ready to help. Over 25 years we shared friendship and activism, and much of what many of us did individually, and with others, was as a direct result of Peter's influence.

In and Out the Bin, and *Doing the Magellan*? I'm astounded, I never knew of either project. But I often thought an autobiography would be wonderful, so publishing what there is, I heartily support.

Louise R. Pembroke, Survivor Activist

0.3

FOREWORD

'There is a pleasure mad men know
Of their kind,
As they embrace at the pot-room door
And the scrutiny of the caring crowd has gone blind.
There is that pleasure then'

That Pleasure, Peter Campbell (2006)

In 2014, I published a historical memoir of what I describe as my mad years (*The Last Asylum: A Memoir of Madness in Our Times*, London: Hamish Hamilton). In the early 1980s I had a breakdown and began what became an intensive psychoanalysis; in the late 1980s I spent four years in mental health institutions, both as an inpatient and day-patient. The 'Last Asylum' of my book's title was Friern Hospital (a huge Victorian pile, known in its heyday as Colney Hatch) where I spent four months in the late 1980s. These were Friern's final years; it closed in 1993.

Writing the book was strange, exciting, sometimes frightening. The task was made easier by people I met while I was researching the history of mental health in Britain. The most memorable of these was Peter Campbell, a leading mental health activist and pioneer of the survivor/user movement.

Peter had much experience of the old asylums, as well as the system of 'care in the community' that replaced them. In 1986 he co-founded *Survivors Speak Out*, the first network organisation, enabling people to work together to share information and campaign for rights and better conditions in hospitals and in the community. He wrote newsletters, advised groups and undertook research. The organisation set a course for user/survivor-led groups, still visible in the National Survivor User Network.

The service-users' movement in Britain began in the early 1970s, when users embroiled in a fracas at the Paddington Day Hospital created a Mental Patients Union (MPU) to take forward their demands.[1] It was the age of radical movements and the MPU was very typical of the times, issuing calls for a 'mad revolution' to accompany the upcoming 'class revolution'. But the specific issues on which the Union campaigned – compulsory detention, the right to refuse treatment, patients' representation on policymaking bodies – were important and urgent, and remained so over the decades as other organizations – *Campaign against Psychiatric Oppression, Survivors Speak Out, the Hearing Voices Network* – emerged and gradually gained a hearing. Voluntary associations acting on behalf of service users (notably Mind) had been important players in the mental health arena for decades, but by the end of the twentieth century they had been joined by a large number of independent service-user groups.

Peter was at the heart of these developments. He was a shy, gentle-mannered man. Meeting him for the first time, I thought him rather timid, an impression that was soon dispelled as I interviewed him and, later, when he contributed to events that I organised. He was a wonderful speaker, never glib but very forceful. When I met him he was nearly deaf but, nonetheless, able to captivate audiences with his wit and devastating accounts of life in the 'bin'. He was also a poet; the opening line of the first poem in his collection *Brown Linoleum Green Lawns* is 'There is a pleasure madmen know'.

In 1986, Peter appeared on television in *We're Not Mad... We're Angry*, a documentary that mixed dramatised sequences scripted by Peter with testimony from people who had been detained in asylums [see 2.02 below]. In the film Peter explained, "If I'm angry, the degree to which I am angry about my treatment is not because I want to tear the system down. It's not because I want to seek vengeance. It's because I see thousands of people like me whose positive contribution to society is being rinsed down the drain." And of course he *was* very angry – as was I. The rage of mental illness, the unbearable frustration, is true for every 'mad' person. "At times it is hard work not to believe we are a separate branch of humanity," Peter said to me. By the time I met Peter, his deafness probably contributed to this, but he handled its difficulties with grace, while at the same time properly expecting interlocutors to accommodate to them.

I was introduced to Peter by his friend, and mine, the psychologist and writer Peter Barham. Peter B knew Peter very well; in a recent exchange, he emphasised to me that Peter's sense that his humanity and credibility had been, and was still being, devalued was the main driver of his reflections, writings and advocacy. Everything that Peter said, and wrote, returns to this theme: the insistence on a recognition of his (and others') compromised humanity. Peter never chose his vocation as a mental health commentator or activist, he had it foisted upon him; his life – his early ambitions and aspirations – were derailed when he was a student at Cambridge and, in the prolonged aftermath, his energies became absorbed in trying to rescue something from the wreckage.

One of the main themes I discussed with Peter was friendship. Friendship and mental illness weren't meant to go together. Before the Second World War, most UK mental hospitals had a policy of breaking up patient friendships by moving one of the friends to an inaccessible ward. The official rationale for this was concern about potential exploitation of vulnerable patients, but the real motives were rather different. They had a 'whiff of conspiracy', Peter said to me. In acute mental health wards staff were overwhelming concerned with maintaining control. Peter recalled being lambasted by a nurse in the 1980s for his friendly support of other patients. When I asked him why the nurse had been so angry he told me the staff thought such relationships made patients 'uppity'. When I repeated this to a woman who had been a charge nurse at Friern, she pointed out to me that friendship between patients threatened the us–them divide between staff and patients. 'Friendship is too normal, it makes the patients seem just like us.' Peter also recalled another incident where he warned nurses about two patients who were going to have a fight. The nurses ignored him; the fight happened and he was called into the nurses' station and berated – 'don't tell us our jobs!'

Not all mental hospitals were like this. Peter spent some time in Fulbourn Hospital in Cambridgeshire which, under the direction of David Clark, was run along 'therapeutic community' lines, replacing hierarchy and control with what was intended as a more patient-led model of treatment. Clark believed that the arbitrary power of the psychiatrist was a huge handicap in dealing with mental illness: 'However relaxed and friendly a doctor might try to be, the fact that he has the power to deny discharge, to order confinement, seclusion or ECT meant that a patient must always be careful of how much he says and how he says it.'

Peter, who was in Fulbourn in 1970, described it to me as the 'best hospital I have ever been in', with daily meetings of the ward 'community', excellent art therapy and drama therapy. His ward was treated as part of Cambridge University for purposes of residence requirement, as so many students were coming there after having breakdowns over examinations and other pressures of college life. This may have been particularly poignant for Peter, having had his own academic career at Cambridge curtailed by mental illness.

Both Peter and I had experience of systemic abuse within the hospitals, although from our conversations it appeared that I had had more than he. Like most women, I had both experienced and witnessed sexual harassment. We had both seen staff maltreating patients, mostly while giving them forcible injections. Both of us saw many patients placed in solitary confinement, sometimes for long periods: an incarceration which Peter viewed as the most damaging abuse in the system.

We spoke at length about the current state of mental health services. 'The social infrastructure has completely gone.' Hospitals were closed, so too were day centres (I knew about these, as I had attended two of them). Isolation and loneliness, poverty, stigmatisation, drugging: all these were commonplace. People with serious problems were being shunted back to general practitioners, with no one to co-ordinate their care, no proper support. 'Community care is built on medication', he told me. There was a huge increase in compulsion: people who refused drugs – delivered to them in their homes by community nurses – were threatened with detainment in mental health centres. The acute wards in these centres were terrible; there was only drugging, no conversation with staff, even his own nurse just ticked boxes. I asked him about MIND, the mental health charity. They 'blab about resilience', he told me, which to him sounded very Victorian.

Had the survivor movement improved things? I thought he would say it had, but no: it had had very limited impact. Its participants were powerless, there were divergent views in the movement with some taking a narrowly reformist line while others, like himself, were more radical. Stigmatisation continued to be a major problem. People were not listening to them; there was no credibility. This affected the whole movement; some people found it intolerable. There had been successes: some good advocacy practices, an end to electrical shock therapy (he was wrong about this: visiting a new mental health centre I saw a room devoted to ECT).

Nonetheless, the survivor movement was still growing, becoming involved with services at every level. Was he still working with it? Not really, he told me, not for six or seven years. He had run out of steam, didn't know people anymore. Peter didn't strike me as a man who had run out of steam but he did seem disenchanted, battle-weary. Yet when I asked him to speak at public meetings I organised after my book's publication he readily agreed and, despite his deafness, delivered talks that were informative, measured, and very moving.

I was immensely saddened to hear of Peter's death, as were many. I hope this book may convey something of his talents, courage, and achievements.

…

Barbara G Taylor, Professor of Humanities, Queen Mary,
University of London

Note

1 Helen Spandler, *Asylum to Action: Paddington Day Hospital, Therapeutic Communities and Beyond* (London, 2006). For the UK service-user movement, see www.studymore.org.uk; Peter Campbell, 'From Little Acorns: The Mental Health Service User Movement', in A. Bell and P. Lindley (eds), *Beyond the Water Towers: The Unfinished Revolution in Mental Health Services, 1985–2005*, Sainsbury Centre for Mental Health (2005), pp. 73–82; Nick Crossley, 'Fish, Field, Habitus and Madness: The First-Wave Mental Health Users Movement in Great Britain', *British Journal of Sociology*, 50:4 (1999), pp. 647–70.

0.4

INTRODUCTION

I have spent a few years of my life in psychiatric asylums. There are many I know who have spent a good few more. But we're here now, in the body of society. This is where we belong. This is where we have always belonged. Here. Not there, in that other place, separated off like curdle.... Out here is where we belong and that is where we're stopping. If the politicians and society don't like it, we'll have to teach them new social skills. No problem!

(Peter Campbell, 1990 [2.10] Numbers in square brackets refer to chapters listed on the contents page)

Setting the scene

This is a book by, and about, a leader of a liberation movement. That movement is the international psychiatric system survivor movement (Wikipedia, 2025). The leader in question is Peter Campbell. Peter was not a remote person, or one who stood on ceremony, so we hope readers will feel comfortable if we address him by his first name. It would be difficult to encounter a less self-important person than Peter. But this is a movement of people more often mocked, vilified and misunderstood than valued or celebrated. Yet they embody some of the most important, intractable and painful problems that can face any of us as human beings. This again may be a reason why a routine response to them has long been to disown and reject them, rather than recognise the overlaps with all of us. If there is a pecking order in human problems, then this one, whether we understand it in terms of madness and distress or psychopathy and mental disorder, must come somewhere near the bottom. Even now, in this context, there sometimes seems to be an essential confusion between punishment and 'treatment', between blame and understanding. The real importance of Peter was, and is, his determination to record and share his own first-hand experience honestly and his pioneering role in this movement. He worked long and hard to make sense of the difficulties that brought him, and so many others within the psychiatric system, and public attention. He worked tire-lessly and collectively with others to bring about positive change in thinking and responses to such difficulties.

The psychiatric system survivor movement was one of the 'new social move-ments' (NSMs) based on identity and lived experience. While there were early manifestations from the 1960s and 1970s (and previous incarnations recorded as far back as the early 1800s), the movement's real emergence tends to be iden-tified as the 1980s. Certainly, that's the time that pioneers like Peter brought it into high visibility. At the heart of it has been people as survivors speaking and acting for themselves. Its development was associated with the establish-ment of local, national and international organisations and networks set up by survivors and centrally involving survivors themselves (Everett, 1994; Wall-craft et al., 2003; Blayney, 2022). It has challenged traditional psychiatric ideas of mental health patients as an isolated group characterised by pathology and deficiency. Instead, it has emphasised the social relations of madness and dis-tress, the barriers and discrimination they face and the need to look beyond the individual for explanations and to treat them in a humanistic and holistic way.

Social movements such as this, going far beyond traditional economistic-based oppositions, have had a transformative effect globally on our daily lives and relations with each other, even if they have often been in unequal struggle with reactionary formal politics. They have been characterised as being based on challenging traditional negative identities imposed on particular people, behaviour and groups. Conspicuous examples are the women's, Black civil rights and LGBTQIA movements, along with the MeToo, Black Lives Matter and Occupy movements. But if many groups facing oppression and discrimina-tion have been fired up by these developments, from indigenous and disabled people, to Gypsies, Roma and travellers, not all have been able to command the same support or visibility. And that has certainly been true of 'mental health service users', which makes the role of Peter Campbell and the issues he fought for all the more important to highlight. If the thrust of traditional understand-ings has often been to marginalise madness and distress as the isolated issues of a damaged minority, what this fresh thinking has done is remind us of the universality of such experience and the importance for all of us of gaining a better understanding of it.

Key contexts

Before introducing Peter Campbell directly, it may be helpful to identify a few key contexts in which to locate this book. Above all, Peter was variously product, beneficiary and critic of the mid-20th century psychiatric revolution that wit-nessed the advent of psychopharmacology and drug treatments and the relocation of the populations of traditional mental hospitals into settings in the community, accompanied by, at the very least, a rhetorical shift in power in favour of ex-patient and family associations, promising those who identified as psychiatric survivors new opportunities, and an expanding role in defining what mental health care should be, and how it should be delivered (Barham, 2020). Here we may highlight:

1 The collective organising of ex-mental patients in the wake of 1968, inspired by the civil rights movement and other NSMs and liberation struggles. The iconic *Madness Network News* was first published in 1972 (Proctor, 2018). For the UK, see Crossley (2005) and Morrison (2005); and for pertinent reflections, see Borch-Jacobsen (2006, 2009).

2 The emergence of new forms of knowledge-making about mad psyches that distance from the 'objective' categories of clinical psychiatry and reach out to the person embedded in a wider, mutable, cultural, social and political context. A classic example is the hearing voices movement which takes voice-hearing out of the realm of psychopathology, relocating it in people's life-problems and personal philosophies (Romme & Escher, 2000). More recently, we have the burgeoning Mad Studies movement (Le Francois et al., 2013; Beresford & Russo, 2021; Jones & Kafai, 2024; Lewis, Ali, & Russell, 2024). These developments are linked to fundamental shifts in outlooks on disabled people from 'objects of welfare and science' to active citizens (Barham, 2021).

3 Critical ethnographic studies of ex-mental patients from the late 1970s and 1980s. A classic study is *Making It Crazy* by Sue Estroff (1981) from Madison, Wisconsin. The mad subjects in Barham's (1991) study of ex-mental patients diagnosed with psychosis in West Yorkshire are more combative than Estroff's subjects, more closely resembling the survivors Peter Campbell mostly engaged with. See also Cohen (2007) and Eghigian (2017). For France, see the important work of the *Groupe Information Asiles* (GIA), the first group ever led by psychiatric users in France, which published a bulletin, '*Psychiatrises en Lutte*', from 1974 to 1979, comprising reports and testimonies by *psychiatrises* (Bernardet, 2008; Henckes, 2021).

4 The vicissitudes of the psyche, and of precarious lives such as those of mental patients, are invariably immersed in the power fields of history (Barham, 2021). The cultural and political resonances of distressed psyches may produce entanglements between psychiatric and political forms of action that can be identified as psycho-politics (Freis, 2019). Reflecting on her own traumatic history, in which she was born in a mental hospital to a white mother, who had been spurned by her family, and a black father, the South African writer Bessie Head concluded that the 'things of the soul' were invariably 'a question of power' (Head, 1974). The physician and anthropologist Didier Fassin argues that precarious lives must be defined not in the absolute of a condition (such as, for instance, in an earlier era of psychiatry, 'constitutional inadequacy') but in relation to those who have power over them (Fassin, 2012). The jurist and mental patient Daniel Paul Schreber, who produced a compelling memoir of his psychosis in 1903, is of special significance here for Schreber insisted that the exposition of his illness was to be read, not simply as an expression of his

personal psychopathology, as his physicians were all too eager to maintain, but also as an expression of an alternative stance within life, and a window onto truths about the society of his period that were generally suppressed or denied (Santner, 1996; Barham, 2021).

Introducing Peter

So, who was Peter Campbell? We can read his biography in his own words shortly in this book, but first a brief account, highlighting the range of his achievements. Though born and raised in the Scottish Highlands, Peter died in London in 2022 at the age of 73, having lived there for most of his adult life. Peter was variously an activist, a writer and a commentator, a long-standing survivor of the mental health system, with a history of multiple hospitalisations, many of them compulsory, starting in 1967, simultaneously a greatly esteemed educator, with honorary doctorates from Anglia Ruskin and from the Open University, and not least a distinguished published poet. A founder and veteran of the groundbreaking psychiatric system survivor movement, he first became prominent during the period in the 1980s and 1990s when mental patients and ex-mental patients in Britain were starting to organise and make their voices heard. He was a key leader of the radical survivor-led organisation *Survivors Speak Out.*

A psychiatric career

In old-fashioned parlance, regarded as stigmatising today, Peter might be described as a 'career psychotic', a designation that he did not entirely eschew, though as an indefatigable critic of orthodox psychiatry, characteristically alluding to 'the difficulties psychiatrists appear to have in combining their role with humanity', he invariably challenged its meanings. His critiques of numerous facets of the mental health system are frequently laced in a mordant wit: 'I have been diagnosed as "manic depressive with schizophrenic tendencies"' he wrote in a letter to the *Guardian* in 1987, 'while this may have helped the experts in prescribing me numerous "drug cocktails" over the years, it has not proved a notable asset on the dance floors of everyday life. One man's diagnostic tool is another three's insult' (*Guardian*, 27 June 1987).

He was a prescient commentator on change in the mental health system, offering a unique service user view and an on-going analysis of the impact of the survivor movement from within. His writing stretches across more than five decades from his first experience of mental distress in 1967 to very near to his untimely death in 2022.

Peter in his own words

At the Heart of a Mad Movement draws together a selection of Peter's key writings and presentations, many of them unpublished. We have been remarkably fortunate to be able to work from his archive and in doing that we have sought to be guided by the diversity of his work and writing, rather than to pre-empt discussion through imposing some narrow selection of our own. At the centre of this collection is an arresting autobiographical critique of psychiatric provision in Britain that Peter wrote between 1983 and 1985, starting from his first breakdown in 1967 just four days into his first term as a history student at Jesus College Cambridge, when he found himself, as he wrote, suddenly 'catapulted from the status of undergraduate scholar to that of long-term mental patient'. Based on the first eighteen years of his career as a mental patient, as he describes it, this memoir has only recently been discovered among his paper and was previously unpublished. Across six chapters, under the title *In and Out the Bin,* it addresses the trajectory of his experience from his first crisis or breakdown, through successive mental hospital admissions to a point where his life, though still routinely punctuated and disrupted by crises and psychiatric hospital admissions, had become more community-centred. Though explicitly intended for publication (Peter submitted it to Pluto Press in 1986 who liked his writing but were not persuaded that the book would work for them commercially (letter from Neil Middleton, 14 March 1986), it has never been published before. In our opinion, it combines invaluable description and analysis, intellect, politics and feeling concerting and enhancing each other, and possesses a vitality and immediacy, even after the lapse of almost 40 years, that will doubtless still touch readers today. At its core is a series of narratives in which Peter relates, and analyses, the disruptions that his experiences of psychosis inflicted upon him; the reactions they stimulated in others, including medical and social services, and how they were dealt with. He relates his struggles, jointly with others in his social milieu, to try to achieve a position in which mental breakdown need not be viewed entirely negatively as 'a caesura and an aberration', but might instead be treated 'as a vital part of a continuing life story'; where mental illness may be seen 'as a process of change, not destruction'; and mental health may be viewed as 'an active developing thing' [1.1].

In the first decades of Peter's mental health career especially, his biography was incessantly punctuated by disruptions, the next crisis already looming on the horizon. 'October 1990 was a bad month for me', he wrote. 'In the course of a single week, I notched up my fourteenth and fifteenth admission into a psychiatric institution'. The field of mental health was never a conscious career choice, or vocation, rather it is where he fetched up, and perforce had to reinvent himself, amidst unfamiliar and sometimes inhospitable surroundings. In the prolonged aftermath of his first breakdown, his energies were slowly absorbed into rescuing something from the wreckage of his previous hopes and ambitions. Trying to 'find new ways to use his personal experience of receiving services and living with a mental illness diagnosis in an educational context'; doing mental health training sessions for the Salvation Army, for instance, by using 'personal histories, personal poetry and discussion' (*Curriculum Vitae 2003*). During this period already, he was remarking on, and finding inspiration in, the growth of the patients' rights and self-advocacy movement, developments that prefigure where his energies would become concentrated in succeeding years.

Key themes

A major theme, which he discusses in numerous commentaries on admissions wards especially, is the impersonality and frequent lack of human connection of the psychiatric system. Another theme is around the concept of breakdown and the meaning of, and provision for, crisis. Does his experience of madness have a meaning or is it something useless, to be rejected? Peter is emphatic about owning and integrating his own madness or distress: 'ultimately, I believe that my distress/madness/psychosis is the real me' [2.16]. He frequently tackles difficult subjects such as seclusion and compulsion but always in a manner that makes them accessible [2.18, 2.19, 3.03, 3.12 and 3.13]. Over the years he wrote extensively for *Open Mind, Asylum Magazine, Mental Health Today* and nursing journals. His writings are frequently ahead of their time, anticipating the problems and possibilities of new developments. We also include some interviews with him that explore in more depth his complex views about psychiatric medication and other matters [3.08, 3.09 and 3.10].

Though Peter was a stern critic of psychiatric orthodoxy, and was always receptive to outlooks and solutions beyond psychiatry, and was consistently hostile to attempts to diminish or disregard the meaning that his experience of psychosis held for him, by no means, however, can his outlook be assimilated into a crude anti-psychiatric position, for he was never in denial about the seriousness of his emotional crises, or about his need for some form (though not necessarily medical) of professional intervention. Indeed, during the 1970s (though not in later years) he often felt that his crises might destroy him. Though he admires those who succeed in doing so, he does not himself incline towards journeying through crisis without medication, instead adopting a pragmatic position in which he values the reassurance that a short-term dose of neuroleptics may bring him out of crisis fairly rapidly [2.16]. Frequently, he succeeds in his writing in maintaining a teasing subtlety and ambiguity in which he never quite denies the existence of mental illness, or his own relation to it, but never quite embraces it either.

The selection in the rest of the collection illustrates the diversity and extent of Peter's contributions and his concerns over the years. In the early 1980s, he gave up any lingering idea of a conventional career and began to address the discrimination facing people with a mental illness diagnosis, writing innumerable pieces over the ensuing three and a half decades, many of them with an autobiographical edge, focusing on issues that were of enduring significance to him, such as seclusion [3.12 and 3.13]; spiritual crisis [2.12]; the experience of psychosis [1.1–1.6, 2.14] and the failings of crisis care [2.11 and 3.05]. Also included are interviews from 2000 and 2005 in which he discusses his experience of ECT, of psychiatric drugs and other topics. Peter is always questioning, setting simplistic analyses in a wider and deeper context, and bringing out suppressed dimensions. He was well-read and knowledgeable, but also consistently modest and unpretentious, communicating, in conversation as in writing, in a clear and uncluttered style that never tries to confuse or overawe anyone.

Speaking for himself

In assembling this collection we have tried as best we can to follow Peter's lead. We have been guided by several principles borrowed from the survivor movement itself. First, we have sought to enable Peter to speak for himself and not speak for him. This principle of self-advocacy lies at the heart of both Peter's work and the survivors' movement. Yet we know from concerns frequently expressed by survivor activists and commentators, that their thoughts and ideas have regularly been analysed and disputed by non-survivor academics and others who seem determined to have the last word. We have aimed to avoid doing that and agreed from early on in the project that our purpose was to enable others to access Peter's writings, not to sit in judgement on him or them, or offer our own critiques and interpretations. Survivors, including Peter, experience enough of that in their lives, without us adding to it. Peter doesn't speak for all survivors and very deliberately makes that clear. But his is a very helpful voice because of the range and depth of his survivor experience and his skill and subtlety in sharing it with us. Not only that, but it is the developing viewpoints and ideas of survivor leaders like Peter that are what is of central importance here. We have sought to avoid mediating them, as much as possible, while recognising that any editor runs the risk of distorting his subject's conclusion and perspective. Though our presentation is set on a scholarly base, we have tried to keep our approach straightforward and accessible, to reach out to a wide range of readers.

Here, we particularly want to highlight the decision we have taken as far as possible not to tinker with, or revise, the text as Peter wrote it in the early 1980s. So, for instance, we have retained all Peter's original headings, even where in some instances they may seem quaint or long-winded. Though Peter can demonstrate a sensitivity to the social context and vulnerability of women to the experience of emotional distress [e.g. 2.02 and 2.13] the text sometimes undoubtedly bears peculiarities, such as the ubiquitous use of the male pronoun, that now feel inappropriate, along with the use of words such as 'looney', 'nutter' and 'dosser' and the use of the verb 'committed suicide', though some of these usages may be intentionally ironic. Regardless of its continuing contemporary relevance, the text is inevitably a product of its period and no doubt, had he been able to review it today, Peter may have wanted at points to reframe some of his claims. There is, however, one habit that we find unacceptable. This is the tendency, familiar in classic psychiatry but embraced also more popularly, to identify the person by the diagnosis, as in 'schizophrenics' or 'manic depressives'. Where Peter falls in with this, as he sometimes does, we have opted for a modified description.

We may briefly highlight the thematic threads that run through the book. We expand on these in the short introductions we have offered to each of the sections as a guide for readers. Loss of control, and the attempt to re-establish that control, were central elements in Peter's life since the age of eighteen. 'By losing control, and having a nervous breakdown, I seemed to have entered a particular dimension of existence which is defined by the fact of its inhabitants' inability to have control, of themselves, their environment, their futures' [2.09]. Aside from exhortations to continue taking the tablets, no advice is ever forthcoming from psychiatric professionals on how to cope with a breakdown. 'To live for eighteen years', he writes in1985, 'with a diagnosed of mental illness, is no incentive for a positive self-image'. The whole psychiatric system is founded on inequality and at times 'it is hard work not to believe that we are a separate branch of humanity" [2.09].

Key insights

However, Peter's experience at the bottom of the pile throws up numerous incentives and pointers, still hugely relevant today, for service user action. Instead of looking vertically to experts as they are encouraged to do, 'we can reach out to those around us who have shared experience' and challenge the widespread belief and stereotypes that the 'mentally ill' are by definition incompetent and inarticulate and dangerous and lacking in insight [2.09]. He wants to locate the content of his crises, and those of other service users, within wider and more creative frameworks such as spirituality and spiritual understanding. 'Telling people that their perceptions in psychosis are meaningless, or have only negative value, places obstacles on the path to spiritual understanding' [2.12]. In contention here are the limitations of an illness model or framework [3.02, 3.08]. 'We would not be breaking any professional codes if we acknowledged that something important was going on in crisis that was not to do with illness. In the acute wards of the next decade, it would be good to see psychosis come out of the shrouds...' [2.16]. The meaning and experience of psychosis tends to be treated dismissively, in Peter's opinion, and not properly acknowledged in its full complexity, existential, epistemological, practical, and political in equal measure [2.14].

Frequently, he has encountered the assertion: 'It's not the real you' [3.06]. 'Spoken sometimes as a comfort, as a control, as a dismissal, this phrase symbolises for me the way mental health workers seek to separate themselves and me from aspects of my distress'. In contrast, 'I have found many, myself included, who believe the capacity for madness is worth integrating into, rather than alienating from, their lives. For us, the declaration "It's not the real you..." is first and foremost an act of therapeutic aggression'. He calls for an extensive re-evaluation of that area of human experience we commonly characterise as mental illness [2.16]. What concerns him most are the spiritual difficulties facing individuals who enter the mental health service system. How do they value their experiences in crises? How do they locate themselves within a society that sees them essentially as damaged and defective human beings? [2.12]. Though he is grateful for the psychiatric dressing station that is the NHS acute psychiatric ward, he also points up its limitations [2.16]. The outstanding issue as he perceives it is something like: can there be created a more effective community in the acute ward through a partnership between mental health workers and users or must the community fragment into individual therapeutic relationships? [2.16]. He regards seclusion as a form of abandonment ('I'm not able to forget the times I have been placed in solitary confinement' [3.13]). Psychiatric services may take him in when he is in crisis, but they frequently seem in his experience of them to disown him. Another poignant and forceful account of crisis admission from 2001, under the pseudonym 'Niall', is *A Barren Experience* [3.05].

The personal is political

The personal and the political, the individual and the collective, are profoundly and intimately connected in Peter's thinking and writing, in which he moves out from the individual to the collective or the communal without leaving the individual behind but, equally, never forgets or neglects the collective when the individual is again in focus. Peter did not approach these questions as a sociological theorist of any kind but as one of a group of mental patients and ex-mental patients, all of whom were struggling to make sense of their situations. For him, 'self-advocacy is the vital element that holds the whole structure together'. Self-advocacy in practice is about collective action for change. 'What has been transforming for me in the last five or six years', he wrote in 1990, 'has been to be part of a collective action. No longer standing in the Charge Nurse's office, an isolated patient, asking for my rights. But working with friends, locally, nationally, internationally, to secure for ourselves what is necessary and rightful'. There are many levels of self-advocacy, right up to the government, but at the root is always and necessarily the individual for 'the critical need is for individuals to be involved in their own treatment and care' [2.10].

Breaking barriers

Peter also experimented with different genres of creative writing. We reproduce here a dramatic script he drafted in 1986 on behalf of a collective of 21 mental health system survivors who produced the groundbreaking Channel 4 Television documentary '*We're not Mad, We're Angry*' and an accompanying commentary that Peter had written, with the intention of submitting it to the *New Statesman* [2.02 and 2.03]. By way of giving a different angle on some of the topics and themes that are discussed more formally, we have also distributed across the book threads from a number of his satirical pieces, and from published letters that he wrote to *OpenMind* magazine, mostly from the 1980s. It is appropriate to emphasise here that Peter valued and experimented with a variety of forms of creative expression and did not privilege one form over another. Until his psychiatric career placed insurmountable obstacles in his path, for quite some years he had envisaged a career working with pre-school children, and simultaneously writing for children, and he achieved a diploma in this sphere. It was entirely characteristic of his outlook that when he decided to approach a literary agent about his writings, he placed his poetry, stories, the dramatic scripts for children he had been writing and the text of *In and Out the Bin*, all in the same basket as co-partners in his creative enterprise.

All three of us as editors knew Peter, Peter Barham and Peter Beresford since the late 1980s. Peter Beresford was a survivor friend and colleague over many years and gave the oration at Peter's funeral. Peter Campbell had nominated Peter Barham as his executor in the event of his death, and after Peter's death in April 2022 he was able to find a home for Peter's extensive archive at the Bishopsgate Institute and to secure funding from the Campbell family for the *Peter Campbell Legacy Project* (PCLP), with Ker Wallwork as project archivist and co-ordinator. The work of the PCLP is on-going, but it has already turned up some remarkable findings including a number of striking pieces that we did not know existed and were unpublished in Peter's lifetime, such as the aforementioned manuscripts for *In and Out the Bin* and *Valuing Psychosis: A Personal View* (1994). The present selection of writings by Peter has been made possible by the creation of the PCLP which, through gathering all of Peter's writing together, has given rich insight into the development of both his creative and campaigning work over the course of his lifetime, from his early experimental fiction and *Marvin Menz* cartoons from the *Survivors Speak Out* newsletters in the 1980s to the rigorous book reviews he published in *OpenMind* and a range of journals in the 2010s.

The breadth and detail of Peter Campbell's extensive archive, compiled over more than four decades, capture important developments in survivors' history providing a nuanced perspective on survivor activism within the political context of historic changes in mental health care and policy, such as the development of care in the community, and changing media and social attitudes towards psychiatric survivors from the 1980s to 2010s, documented through an extensive collection of press cuttings. The work of a range of collaborative survivor organisations are documented in Peter's archives including *Survivors Speak Out*, *Camden Consortium* and cross-organisational collaborative campaigning against ECT from the 1990s, as well as Peter's efforts to galvanise campaigning work through the development of a shared survivor perspective on the use of psychoactive medications.

Peter's emphasis on collaboration and consensus building are also demonstrated in his sensitive and rigorous educational work, particularly regarding advocacy and the training of approved social workers, nurses and clinical psychologists. Despite his personal experiences of harm from the psychiatric system and the entrenched power imbalance, the archives demonstrate Peter's generosity and dedication to working constructively and collaboratively, drawing on his own experience to engender empathy and improve the treatment of those in crisis.

Peter Campbell's archives will be a tremendous resource for all those interested in the survivor movement and its history and will link with other survivor history collections, notably Anne Plumb's *Ear to the Ground, Survivor/Service User/Mad Identified (SSUMI+) and Ally Voices, Organisations and Action in the UK, 1971–2010* catalogue, available online http://tinyurl.com/eartotheground with material on loan to Archivesplus in the Central Library in Manchester; Tower Hamlets African and Caribbean Mental Health Organisation (THAC-MHO) archives at Tower Hamlets Local History Library & Archives; and the papers collected by Peter's close colleague and friend Andrew Roberts whose 'Survivor Archives' from the 1970s to early 2020s are already available for researchers' use at the Bishopsgate Institute in London.

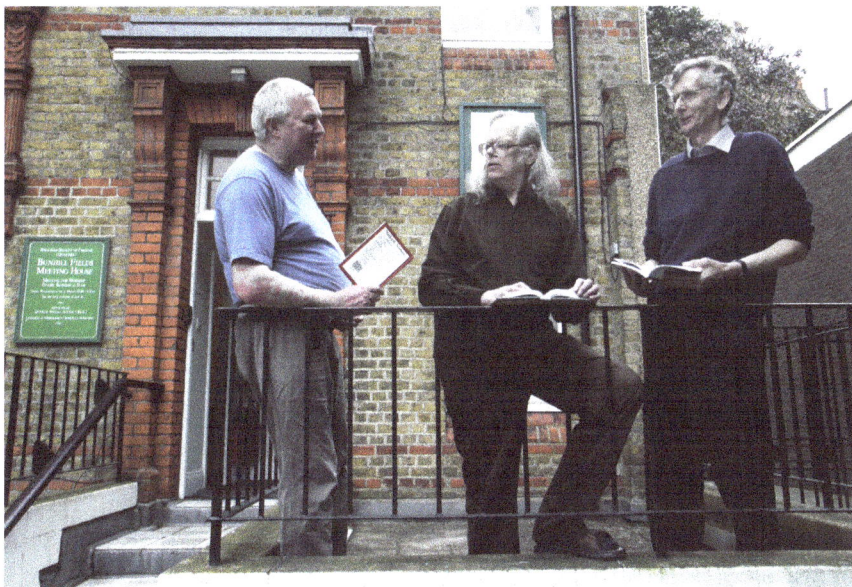

Photograph by Frank Baron, Copyright The Guardian

Enduring insights

It will be clear from the summary of the material that has already been assembled in the PCLP that the present selection of Peter's writings and presentations is by no means exhaustive or comprehensive or does full justice to Peter's overall contribution as a thinker, writer and activist, and if desired there is ample scope among the papers in the PCLP archive for another Campbell collection in the future. In the meantime, we hope that the present book will succeed in conveying the quality of Peter Campbell's thought and writing, his humanity and sensitivity and the forceful perspective he brings to the key development of a new survivor movement that tends to be neglected and given low priority. Even though the psychiatric system changed over the decades in which Peter was a mental patient, much of what he writes, across a diversity of topics and concerns, sadly still holds, and continues to possess an immediacy. This is perhaps a harsh reflection on the inadequacy of official responses to madness and distress. Peter had a gift of identifying the enduring issues and getting to people's core concerns. Many of the issues he raised have not yet been resolved or even adequately addressed. He gives voice to a highly distinctive outlook on what it means to have lived with a diagnosis of psychosis over several decades, all the while playing a combative role in challenging prevailing shibboleths and practices around madness/mental health. His achievement is to bring a wholly original slant to the whole topic area of post-war psychiatry, madness and distress that may also throw light on the era itself. He does in his book as he did it in the movement and in his life. Taken together, this material is a massive indictment of modern psychiatry-based mental health systems and services, which have shown a massive capacity to resist progressive change, and, above all, a testimony to the humanity, unflagging commitment and staying-power of a hugely significant innovator, commentator and critic, with a nuanced voice, who was always honestly upfront in what he said.

Survivors are often stereotyped as isolated and lonely figures, 'loners' and victims of family and social breakdown. This is a reductive concept that flattens the complex and varied reality of survivors' lives and denies the collaborative and communal work that many are involved in and is documented in this book. Thus, Peter was a very social and sociable person, with strong, long-standing friendships and great skills in working and collaborating with others. He was a people person, in that sense, who worked collaboratively both with other survivors and professionals and built strong friendships (Jones et al., 2024). This is important because there are serious limits to what isolated activism can achieve and, whatever difficulties he faced, from early on Peter adopted a different, much more collective and inclusive approach to what is ultimately a social as well as a personal concern. However, being an activist is no easy road, especially when linked with the kind of difficulties and barriers that a mental health service user/survivor can face on a daily basis. Peter was a tall fit person. As he reports, he had direct experience of physical and verbal abuse as a psychiatric system survivor. He sometimes said that if had been Black he wondered if he would have survived in the psychiatric system with its routine racism and violence. His life as a mental patient spanned the shift from simplistic assumptions about psychiatric disorder to new thinking about Mad Studies, but in a Western psychiatric system still much more closely tied to the former, if we are honest with ourselves. Psychiatry has shown itself a powerful force with an enormous capacity to resist change. That's another reason why insights and experience of people like Peter continue to be invaluable. Our only regret is that some of his most significant writings were not published in his lifetime, and that, overall, many of his scattered writings are relatively inaccessible. We hope now that by bringing together a selection of key writings they can have their fullest impact in a world that seems ever more maddening.

Peter's writing and experience offer a sharp warning that we should be wary of accepting the current conventional wisdom that mental illness is no different to physical ill health and should be regarded in the same way. This is clearly an unhelpful assumption, but if we are to develop more holistic understandings of our wellbeing, then Peter's reportage offers a forcible and timely reminder that much rethinking needs to be done and policy informed by different, kinder premises and understandings.

We end here with Peter Campbell's poem, *The Mental Marching Band*, which he frequently performed himself at festivals and conferences and envisages an alternative future to the one preferred by the psychiatric establishment for the community of psychiatric service users:

You'd better wet your whistles
For the Mental Marching Band
For we're making a wee comeback
And it's spreading through the land.
And we'd laugh you to distraction
If we thought you'd understand
About the Mental Marching Band.
There's Danny Ogenkenyu
On the bagpipes by the way.
And when he's took his Lithium
Sweet Jesus can he play.
You can denigrate the madness
The song won't fade away
From the Mental Marching Band.
We'll all be out and running
When the storm breaks.
Down the House of Commons
Wi' our fruitcake
You'll have to take your medication then
Just for the music's sake
And the Mental Marching Band
We'll not be taking prisoners
Under blood red skies.
We've had too much confinement
In our lives.
We're getting our own World War out
That everyone survives.
Thanks to the Mental Marching Band.
Let's hear it.
            [From: Peter Campbell, *Brown*
                Linoleum Green Lawns,
                    Hearing Eye 2006]

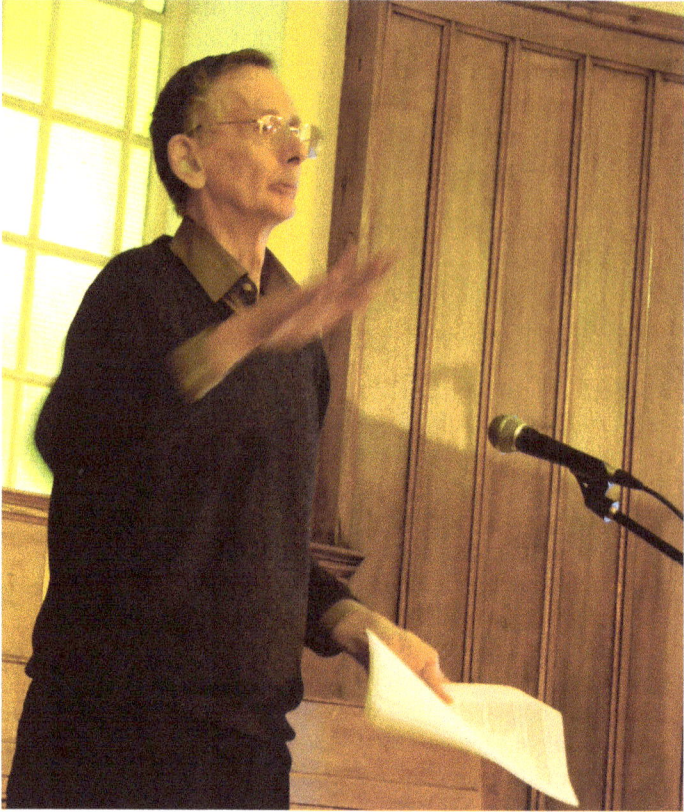

References

Barham, Peter (2021) 'The Mental Patient in History', in: D. McCallum ed., *The Palgrave Handbook of the History of Human Sciences.* London: Routledge.

Barham, Peter (with Hayward, Robert) (1991) *From the Mental Patient to the Person*, London: Routledge.

Barham, Peter (2020) *Closing the Asylum: The Mental Patient in Modern Society*, London: Penguin Books, 1992; second edition 1997; third edition 2020, with a new prologue and a preface by Peter Campbell, London: Process Press Ltd.

Beresford, Peter & Russo, Jasna eds. (2021) T*he Routledge International Handbook of Mad Studies*, London: Routledge.

Bernardet, Philippe (2008) 'Apercu historique du G.I.A. De 1972 a 1992', in: Nicole Maillaird-Dechenans ed., *Pour en Finir avec la Psychiatrie: Des patients temoignent*, St Georges d'Oleron: Les Editions Libertaires.

Blayney, Steffan (2022) 'Activist Sources and the Survivor Movement', in: Chris Millard and Jennifer Wallis eds, *Sources in the History of Psychiatry, from 1800 to the Present*, London: Routledge

Borch-Jacobsen, Mikkel (2006) 'Usagers de therapies et producteurs de maladies. Breves remarques historico-speculatives sur l'etat present du champ "psy"', www.ethnopsychiatrie.

net, 'Les textes du colloque des 12 et 13 Octobre 2006, "La Psychotherapie a l'Epreuve de ses Usagers"'.

Borch-Jacobsen, Mikkel (2009) 'Therapy Users and Disease Mongers', in: *Making Minds and Madness: From Hysteria to Depression*, Cambridge: Cambridge University Press.

Cohen, Bruce M.Z. (2007) *Mental Health User Narratives*, London: Palgrave Macmillan.

Crossley, Nick (2005) *Contesting Psychiatry; Social Movements in Mental Health*, London: Routledge.

Eghigian, Greg ed. (2017) *The Routledge History of Madness and Mental Health*, London: Routledge.

Estroff, Sue (1981) *Making it Crazy*, Berkeley, Calif.: University of California Press.

Everett, Barbara (1994) 'Something Is Happening: The Contemporary Consumer and Psychiatric Survivor Movement in Historical Context', *The Journal of Mind and Behaviour*, 15 (1 and 2), pp. 55–70. https://www.brown.uk.com/brownlibrary/EVERETT.htm accessed 26 January 2025.

Fassin, Didier (2012) *Humanitarian Reason: A Moral History of the Present*, Oakland: University of California Press.

Freis, David (2019) *Psycho-Politics between the World Wars: Psychiatry & Society in Germany, Austria and Switzerland*, London: Palgrave Macmillan.

Head, Bessie (1974) *A Question of Power*, London: Heinemann Educational.

Henckes, Nicolas (2021) 'Negotiating the Limits of Therapy: Patients', Families', and Nurses' Perspectives on Therapeutic Failure in the Aftermath of the Psychiatric Revolution, 1970s–1980s', *Medizinhistorisches Journ* 1, 56 (1–2), pp. 79–102.

Jones, Melanie & Kafai, Shayda eds. (2024) *Mad Scholars: Reclaiming and Reimagining the Neurodiverse Academy*, New York: Syracuse University Press.

Le Francois, Brenda, Menzies, Robert, & Reaume, Geoffrey (2013) *Mad Matters: A Critical Reader in Canadian Mad Studies*, foreword by Peter Beresford, Toronto: Canadian Scholars Press.

Lewis, Bradley, Ali, Alisha, & Russell, Jazmine eds. (2024) *Mad Studies Reader*, London: Routledge.

Morrison, Linda (2005) *Talking Back to Psychiatry: The Psychiatric Consumer/Survivor/Ex-Patient Movement*, London: Routledge.

Plumb, Anne (2022) *Ear to the Ground: Catalogue of a Personal Archive Collection in Mental Health (1971-2010) - Survivor, Service User, Mad Identified, and Ally Voices*, Manchester: TBR Imprint; tinyurl.com/eartotheground

Proctor, Hannah (2018) 'Mad World: Radical Psychiatry and 1968', Verso Blogpost, 19 June 1018.

Roberts, Andrew, Mental Health History Timeline, http://studymore.org.uk accessed 6 February 2025.

Romme, Marius & Escher, Sandra (2000) *Making Sense of Voices: A Guide for Mental Health Professionals Working with Voice-Hearers*, London: MIND Publications.

Santner, Eric (1996) *My Own Private Germany: Daniel Paul Schreber's Secret History of Modernity*, Princeton University Press.

Wallcraft, Jan, Read, Jim, & Sweeney, Angela (2003) *On Our Own Terms: Users and Survivors of Mental Health Services Working Together for Support and Change*, London: The Sainsbury Centre for Mental Health https://survivorresearcher.net/resources/ accessed 26 January 2025.

Wikipedia (2025), Outline of the Psychiatric Survivors Movement, https://en.wikipedia.org/wiki/Outline_of_the_psychiatric_survivors_movement accessed 26 January 2025.

0.5

PETER INTRODUCES HIMSELF: c 2005

Peter Campbell was born and brought up in the Scottish Highlands. In 1967, he went down to England to study at university and almost immediately was admitted into a psychiatric unit. Between 1967 and 1972, he was in four different hospitals (two in Scotland, two in England), before graduating and ending up in one of the 'Epsom Cluster' asylums for a year. He then moved to London, where he lived in a therapeutic community in the Ladbroke Grove area, and came in contact with COPE, an offshoot of the Mental Patients Union. He did not get actively involved at this point.

For most of the next ten years, Peter was on the 'bed-sitting room circuit' in North-West London, attempting to build a career, first working with preschool children (not something a 'psychotic' male would have much joy with in the 1990s) and then as a bookseller. In the early 1980s, he gave up any idea of a conventional career and began to address the discrimination facing people with a mental illness diagnosis. He began to work regularly as a 'volunteer' with Mind in Camden. At this time, there were very few independent service user groups. Peter was involved with CAPO (*Campaign Against Psychiatric Oppression*), although he was never a member, and *British Network for Alternatives to Psychiatry*, which had links to David Cooper and R.D. Laing and was a mixture of survivors and mental health workers. In the mid-1980s, ideas of advocacy and service user involvement had barely emerged.

Peter was one of the first survivor members of *Camden Mental Health Consortium*, a group growing out of the concern about closure plans for Friern Barnet hospital that became one of the earliest local service user-led groups. In 1986, he was a founder member of *Survivors Speak Out* and continued to be actively involved, often as an officer of the organisation, until 1996. In 1991, he and three other survivor poets that he had first met through CAPO poetry and music events founded *Survivors' Poetry*. Around about the same time, Peter began to earn a living as a freelance writer and trainer in the mental health field, a job that he continues at the present time. He continues to receive mental health services as an inpatient and outpatient.

Fifteen years on, Peter wonders whether service user organisations are not too closely involved in mental health services. To what extent have groups attempted to address the general public rather than mental health workers? Why has the "user movement" done so little to work with other oppressed groups? Why is our record of action on civil rights issues (unless they're part of Mental Health Act changes) so poor? Why have service user survivor organisations always found it so difficult to communicate and work with each other?

Peter's greatest fear – that people with a mental illness diagnosis will be seen as a special type of disabled citizen whose social inclusion depends upon good behaviour and complying with a programme of activities and treatment.

Greatest hope – that the general public get to hear about, and appreciate, the achievements of collective action by service users/survivors.

Important tip – if you don't enjoy service user action, get out of it and find something you do enjoy…

IN AND OUT THE BIN, 1967–85

1.00a

INTRODUCTION TO PART 1, *IN AND OUT THE BIN*, 1967–85

Part 1 comprises Peter's autobiographical narrative under the title *In and Out the Bin,* which he composed between 1983 and 1985 to describe and critically examine his experience between 1967, the time of his first breakdown, and the mid 1980s, the time he was writing. We have already summarized the scope of this narrative in the introduction, and it is conveyed in more detail in Peter's own synopsis, narrated in the first person, which follows this note.

Several chapters listed in the synopsis, namely Six, Seven, Nine, Ten, Eleven and the appendix, were never completed, though they all treat themes that Peter addressed in subsequent writing. Chapter 8 in the synopsis, 'Drugs-The Many-Headed Guard Dog', is now Chapter 6 [1. 06] Though it is illuminating to be able to grasp the scope of the project as Peter had originally envisaged it, the kernel of the book is undoubtedly fulsomely conveyed in the existing chapters [1. 01–1. 06] In Chapter 2 [1. 02], we become aware of how Peter is being radicalised, identifying with the have-nots rather than the haves, as he puts it, and finding himself in, and embracing, an outsider position. In Chapter 3 [1. 03] the breakdown experience itself assumes a special salience and Peter expatiates at some length on his struggles to win control of his own breakdown process and on the distortion, perversion even, of the breakdown experience as he witnesses it, and of the meaning of breakdown, in the social and clinical environment in which he was immersed. In Chapter 5 [1. 05], the benefit of a sojourn in a therapeutic community introduces Peter to a realm completely at odds with the world of the traditional mental hospital with which he had heretofore mostly been familiar and the dawning recognition that mental illness need not actually be the wholly negative experience that he had been led to suppose over so many years.

DOI: 10.4324/9781003636434-2

1.00b

PETER'S SYNOPSIS OF "IN AND OUT THE BIN"

We have included Peter's Synopsis for 'In and Out the Bin' so readers may appreciate the scope of the book as Peter originally envisaged it. Note, however, that some of the envisaged chapters were never completed and as a result the numbering of the chapters in the present book diverges from the numbering in Peter's synopsis. From 1.01 onwards we reproduce the fully completed chapters that make up the central core of 'In and Out the Bin'.

In and Out the Bin is an autobiographical critique of N.H.S. psychiatric provision and a description of the quality of life experienced by an individual with mental health problems in contemporary Britain. It concentrates on the effect of the psychiatric process on the individual rather than detailing the inner world of "madness", red in tooth and claw. It aims to show mental illness as a process of change, not destruction, and to highlight the areas where current attitudes, in society and in hospital, prevent the individual's life progress and diminish his status.

In and Out the Bin is firmly based on my own personal experience. It is an attempt to prove that reasoned criticism of psychiatry from a recipient without professional expertise is possible and that an individual's life experience of "mental illness" need not be either anecdote or sensation. It attempts to show the common problems faced by the ordinary person and the ordinary "nutter", as well as the special problems the latter may face "In and Out the Bin".

Chapter One: Introduction

The book is an account based on *personal* experience. The peculiar advantages and limitations of such a perspective. Some indication of how attempts to write my "life story" and a consumer's guide to psychiatric services both proved unsatisfactory. Reasons why I have avoided descriptions of the internal world of "madness". Essentially divisive in effect. The great terminology debate – mentally ill?, consumers?, users?, recipients?, system survivors? Author's choice. Use of male gender explained.

DOI: 10.4324/9781003636434-3

Chapter One: First Taste [1.01]

(Autobiographical). This chapter details the course of my first breakdown and admission, on arrival at Cambridge University in 1967. It includes a short account of my childhood and schooling to indicate the impact breakdown had upon me.

I describe my first reactions to a psychiatric ward and then indicate some of the common elements of in-patient life on a psychiatric ward.

Chapter Two: Cambridge--The Golden Land [1.02]

(Autobiographical). This chapter follows my five years and two further breakdowns while at Jesus College, Cambridge. How I moved from a position of loner to complete outsider and how great a role "mental illness" played in this change. How eventually I was separated from the expectations of my peers.

This chapter also includes comment on the supposedly cataclysmic nature of descents into madness, the importance of behaviour as a measure of mental illness and the difficulties psychiatrists appear to have in combining their role with humanity.

Chapter Three: Breakdowns and Shakedowns [1.03]

(Critique). An analysis of breakdown and admission. The practical and symbolic importance of breakdown to the victim. The difficulties facing an individual in throes of breakdown: lack of choice, ignorant general practitioners (GPs), inappropriate facilities. Does seeking help make you worse? Breakdown as an experience to suffer not to participate in. The mental patient's supposed lack of insight – is it merely an excuse founded on convenience? Do professionals really want to involve patients in their own breakdowns? Breakdown as a loss of power. Psychiatric process confirms that loss.

I include examples from my own experience, illustrating drugging out, undifferentiated response to differing degrees of crisis. Whose best interests are served by current practice? My own impression that my self-discovery was obstructed by the attitudes of N.H.S. carers.

Chapter Four: Life on the Inside [1.04]

(Critique). Impressions of life on an admission ward. The nature of in-patient experience and how it has changed since the 1940s. Changeable nature of ward life – fluctuations of mood and membership. Psychiatric games-playing from the trivial to the oppressive pursuit. Playing games games; we are observing you games; democratic ward meeting games.

The balance of power and its abuses. Why do mental patients have such negative feelings about the ward experience? Life on the inside as a reflection of realities on the outside.

Chapter Five: Therapeutica-Chinks in the Armour [1.05]

(Autobiographical). A year in a Richmond Fellowship therapeutic community. An important turning point. Interruption in a career as "patient". Description of community life and processes and its major differences from a psychiatric unit. Ways in which the community helped and failed to help me.

Mid-1970s as a blossoming of alternative and humanistic therapies. A choice of world pictures. Personal experiences in encounter, gestalt and bioenergetic groups. Benefits and limitations. Growth of a belief that I might really be able to take control of my life.

Chapter Six: Dance of the Revolving Door

(Autobiographical). Coming to terms with life as a manic-depressive. The effects of recurrent breakdown upon my attempts to live a normal life. How do you "sell" mental illness to your friends and lovers? A description of the revolving door syndrome as I experienced it and the possibility that it can be a learning experience and not a sterile choreographed routine.

My increasing understanding of the day-to-day situations which could precipitate crises. The growing belief that I would not be destroyed by manic episodes. The argument that people can learn from experiences as well as analysis. The need for agencies to intervene and help the individual to jam the revolving door.

Chapter Seven: Doctors and Nurses

(Critique). The relationships which exist between the professionals in the caring team and the recipient of psychiatric services. The limitations the system imposes upon the professional – the conflict between professional and human responses. My own experience of psychiatrists – the handicap of limited time; the handicap of different cultural and linguistic backgrounds; inflexibility; the psychiatrist's need to remain in control of transactions; the individual, hostage in another's world picture.

My own experience of nursing staff, in particular the effect of staff shortage in limiting their role to that of administrators and custodians. Occupational therapists, social workers and psychologists. Occupational therapists and psychologists as the unrealised potential within the system. My own encouraging experiences of occupational therapy, and the possibilities for positive activity-based "treatment" for mental health problems. How much are we masters of the system, how much the victims? Is the emotional environment right?

Chapter Eight: Drugs-The Many-Headed Guard Dog [1.06]

(Critique). An analysis of the positive and negative effects of the chemotherapy revolution and the current dominant position of drug therapies in N.H.S. psychiatry.

A historical outline of the changes in mental health experience since the discovery and first use of chlorpromazine. The undoubted benefits. Outline of the reactions to chemotherapy in mid-1970s and 1980s. The dangers. Chemotherapy in the context of no effective alternative therapies. Dependence of recipient. Dependence of professional on drug-orientated philosophies. Staff hypocrisy and double standards.

Personal experiences of N.H.S. drug culture. Labelled as anti-drug. Behaviour seen as a result of supposed compliance or non-compliance in drug use. Total absence of information regarding the possibilities of drugs and their side-effects. Use of dis-information in this area. Freedom without choice – is it possible? The methods of dispensing drug treatments as damaging as possible side-effects. N.H.S. dependence on drugs as an economic and convenience strategy linked to goals – e.g., rapid return to community – which are unconvincing in human terms. The possibilities of an approach based on the needs of the individual.

Chapter Nine: Treatments and Mistreatments

(Critique). Consideration of some of the more controversial treatments: E.C.T.; locked wards; padded cells. "Compulsion" in a caring environment.

Discussion of E.C.T. can be the unpleasantness of treatment, the psychological damage it causes, be justified in the light of the doubtful degree of its successful use? E.C.T. as a sword of Damocles. Compulsion and E.C.T. Is E.C.T. necessary?

Is it possible to found a caring service upon compulsion? The direct and indirect effects of compulsory treatment as a possibility in psychiatric care. The effect upon staff attitudes. The absurdities inherent in the current use of sectioning.

The necessity of locking patients up. Personal experience of this. Set against the above need is the use of locked wards as a logistic and man-management device. The danger that compulsion is abused in order to maintain the subordinate status of the mental patient, regardless of the real needs of the situation. Why do so many ex-patients feel punished? Are they being covertly punished?

Chapter Ten: One Step Forward and Duck

(Autobiographical). Mental health and employment. An account of how mental health problems affected and did not affect my career. Some of the obvious handicaps recurrent illness imposed. Working with Under-5s in Inner London. Being advised to give up this work and look for different employment. Return to Under-5s. Proving the experts wrong. Pressures of past forcing me towards self-employment.

Employers and mental illness. Learning to lie at interviews. Refusing to lie at interviews. The many cruel employers, the few who will give you a chance. Ignorance and hypocrisy in the 1970s. Impossibilities in the 1980s. Refusing to accept the shame. Employment and self-worth – the prices of capitalism.

Total inadequacy of support for ex-patients needing work. Why do we stop at occupational therapy? The Disablement Officer – "I'm quite sure I can't help you, you know". The limitations inherent in current concepts of employment. The psychiatric promise as a badly constructed con-trick.

Chapter Eleven: Well Out the Bin

(Critique/Autobiographical). Living successfully in the community. Growth of the Patients' Rights/Self-Advocacy movement.

The positive aspects. Possibility of seeing mental health as an active developing thing. My personal response to my own career as a manic-depressive. My current life and lifestyle.

The need to acknowledge the equal value of the recipient's experience. The belief that the ability of human beings to help each other in crisis exists, but is currently dissipated by institutional forms.

Description of Patients' Rights growth. Conclusion.

Appendix: An Account of One Episode of "Madness" – October 1971.

Reconstruction of internal and external world of a manic episode, with some commentary and remarks on "madness" negative and positive.

1.01

"FIRST TASTE"

I awoke in the early hours of the morning. The glow of the city lit the window. Something had happened. Something had changed and I was afraid. I had been asleep for three or four hours and dreamed the most disturbing dreams. In fact, the stream of images had been so vivid and so continuous in my mind that it was hard to believe that I had been asleep at all. It was like a particular, cogent hallucination, a fever of the brain. I have only experienced such a thing on two or three occasions since and then always while under the influence of a particular tranquilising drug. But this was the first time and I was stone-cold sober. It was immediately very frightening, sitting on the bed in that darkened room while the realities of my imagination resolved and failed to resolve themselves within me. My stomach turned with an uncertain fear that did not respond to reason. Eventually I was calm – to the extent that I was aware of my separate existence and that of the washbasin and the gas-fire. The hierarchies of reality established themselves; the priorities were restored. But inside that re-discovered calm a greater fear had begun. One cannot always efface with reason what is truly felt. For I was different. Something had indeed changed. A hole appeared which now could never disappear.

Is it possible to go mad overnight? Normally such a notion would seem to belong only to ghost and horror fiction or to Gothic romance. But on a passage from sanity to madness, or from normality to mental illness, there must come a point in time when an individual crosses the line. It has been customary for society, nowadays chiefly in the guise of experts, to dictate at what point such a crossing occurs and to festoon that decision with the long streamers of antecedents and prior causation. It has become customary for many mentally ill (some would say it is part of their situation) to claim that they have not yet crossed that line past which they have been prematurely pushed, or to complain that society keeps shifting the frontiers around to suit its own purposes. These are reflections of social and political realities. But there is a personal dimension. I believe many individuals do reach a moment when they clearly recognise madness within themselves. Everyone acknowledges such a phenomenon within themselves in a theoretical sense. It is on such fearful recognition that much prejudice against the mentally ill is founded. But to feel madness as a tangible part of you, or as a concrete potential within you, is an experience of

DOI: 10.4324/9781003636434-4

a completely different order. To feel and acknowledge this need not be the same as being mad or going mad. It may be the recognition of a new relationship within you to the irrational, or the possibility of interruption in your contact with the real world. Or the feeling in the pit of your stomach that all is not what it used to seem. It is a moment of recognition. Thus, although when I arose that following morning I had in no way become mad, indeed, was subsequently diagnosed to be suffering from mere anxiety neurosis, I had in fact during the course of one night passed a significant junction to which it is not possible to return. Although I was still myself, I was also something other.

That night-time discovery was a heavy blow. There I was an eighteen-year-old ex-public schoolboy only four days into my first term at Cambridge University and already coming apart at the seams. The reasons for my dramatic change in fortunes, my increasing self-separation from the new environment I had entered were not apparent to me at the time. Indeed, it was not until much later that I began to ask the question – why me? Immediately the unexpectedness of events was paramount.

Childhood is a sacred place to many who are no longer children. Mental patients can rarely afford such a luxury. Most of us have had our childhoods ploughed, raked and harrowed by the questions of psychiatrists, to the extent that we feel easier and less guilty if we can produce evidence of unhappiness as a child than if we cannot. But if I pull out a selection of picture cards from the sack of memory and an expert arranges them to make me blame my mother, what kind of truth may that be – either to me or to childhood? It is not always easy to form one's childhood into the clear path of an explanation. Nor to mould it around the spine of another's theory. Unfortunately, matters are further complicated by the fact that not everyone ploughs the field of childhood in the same direction. The Freudian expert may go north to south and ensure a deep furrow while the humanistic psychotherapist may go east-west for less landslip and better drainage. They are probably both right. But for the fields of our childhoods such differing methods can cause considerable erosion. I believe everyone wishes to protect their childhood memories no matter how tenuous the connection between memory and truth may be.

It is not childhood's prime function to serve as explanation. But the psychiatrist's armoury is based on questions. Certainly answering questions is inherent in the role of mental patient. Many clients build up defences against such probings. I am sure that somewhere in the course of the last fifteen years I acquired a story of my childhood which was at once suitable for an audience trained in psychiatry and yet sufficiently untrue for me to retain my own mystery intact. It is not such an account nor an attempt at explanation that follows. To a degree my childhood remains sacred. The details I include are only intended to provide a sketch by which to better judge the impact of my first breakdown.

I was born on 3 January 1949 in the village of Strathtay on the banks of the River Tay. I am the youngest of three brothers. As children we were independent and self-contained and adulthood has not altered those distances between us. My father was an ornithologist and his passion dictated that we should be brought up among the mountains of the Scottish Highlands. Our summer holidays were most often spent on the west coast of Scotland or among the even greater loneliness of the Outer Hebrides, my father's particular territory. When I was seven and a half, I went to a preparatory school just outside Pitlochry – a small town about five miles from home, and subsequently at thirteen to a public school Trinity College, Glenalmond, on the edge of the Highlands north-west of Perth. At both schools I followed in my brothers' footsteps. Before I went to public school we moved home to the hills above Blairgowrie in eastern Perthshire where my father had purchased two farms. Although my upbringing, isolated in the midst of the Scottish countryside, has affected me greatly, I was not as a child an "outdoor" type. I loved hill-walking and often explored the moors around our estate on my own, but I never became involved in the hunting and fishing rituals common in that rural society. I remember spending much time indoors during holidays, reading and writing stories. The countryside was a background to my imagination rather than an integral part of it.

Public school was very much my social outlet. Like everyone else who has started boarding school at the age of seven and a half I spent far more of my formative years in educational institutions than I did within the institution of the family. I enjoyed public school greatly and academically I was successful. The rampant homosexuality and sadism which so many film-makers and playwrights have detected in the public school system were not a feature of my private education. Indeed, in general we tended much more to stodginess and complacency. It was the era of the Beatles, the Stones and the off-shore pirate radio stations. Teenage rebellion was a commodity seized on by commercial interests and broadcast throughout Britain. Although we were by no means immune to the teenage revolution, I do not believe our attitudes were much affected while at school. The revolution was one of style rather than substance. Our rebellions against the adult world and the authority structure in the public school system were always muted by our essentially middle-class and conservative outlook. For myself with little or no access to the urban cultures where many of my school-friends had their homes, rebellion was only token. Protest was not the leitmotif of my teens. In retrospect the most striking elements of public school I remember are the numerous petty and often quite pointless rules and customs and the unabashed ease with which we accepted them.

As I approached my first day at Cambridge University, I was very much a product of the system with which I had lived. Academically inclined, I was conservative in outlook and marked by my upper-middle class background. The boundaries of my view of the world were firmly fixed and the view itself ordered by the complacency of assumed success. I was converted to the idea that hard work and success were different sides of the same coin. At no point had I considered that one day I might find myself deposited on the outer side of these boundaries. My outlook assumed that the boundaries themselves would naturally expand to always accommodate the progress of my life and career. The idea that something was going to go badly wrong simply never occurred.

By the morning of my fourth day at the university, I could no longer avoid the fact that things were falling apart. The experience of the previous night, although not tenable in the face of rational examination, had undermined my ability and now fed my anxieties. After breakfast I sought out the college chaplain. He tried to calm me but my fears were running out of control. Unconsciously I think I had already perceived the ultimate destination and was now hastening towards it. During the course of the day, my anxiety began to attach itself to completely irrelevant subjects and objects. My sense of being lost in a strange land of hidden and half-understood traps, of being alone in a new world whose rules I had not learnt was, in retrospect, probably shared by a number of the other new undergraduates. But the severity of my reaction was individual and rapidly carried me into an unreal relation to, or isolation from, the immediate environment. By the late afternoon of that day I was completely overcome. Surprisingly, the extent to which I had shrunk away from a proper relationship did not appear to be immediately obvious to those who came into contact with me. I had decided that the only solution was some kind of physical removal from the problem and became afraid that this was not going to be achieved. Finally, the chaplain took me to see a psychiatrist. She interviewed me and then spoke to the chaplain while I waited outside. When I was called in again, she suggested that I return to college that night with some pills to calm me. It was a terrible moment. Somehow, I persuaded her to admit me to a hospital. It was the first, and almost only, occasion on which I have talked myself into the bin.

In fact, it was not a true bin at all, but an annexe of Addenbrooke's hospital that I had entered. I have only fragmentary memories of the next few days there, and they are all unpleasant. If I had thought I would find asylum, I was mistaken. My anxiety fed upon itself. I was worried about being worried. It is not easy to describe acute anxiety. It has a drumming insistence which reduces you to incoherency. I think I became much as a distressed child. I remember trying to smother myself in my pillows and even beating my head against the walls of my room. It was a most unfunny time. I was also shocked by the nature of what had happened to me, and by the unexpected and unwanted potentials that had been revealed as mine. The spectre of failure began to attach itself to my illness. Whether or not I characterised this as a nervous breakdown at the time I cannot now say, but the sheer unexpectedness of this experience, the fact that it lay completely beyond the horizons of my expectations distressed me greatly. Thus the symptoms were aggravated. My anxiety was so great that I could not understand what was being said on the radio headphones, nor attempt the simple jigsaw a therapist left me. I felt I was disintegrating and that my life was finished.

It was decided to transfer me back to the mental hospital in Scotland nearer to my parents. They came down to accompany me back. But a complication had arisen. I had been given barbiturates since my admission and I now proved to be allergic to them. The major effect of this was that my joints seized up so that I could not walk. As a result, I went home to Scotland on a stretcher. My conviction that I was on the scrapheap grew during that journey. My inability to walk, although explained to me, merely underlined my sense of affliction. I remember asking if I was being taken away to die. This was certainly my belief. The shame and other moral implications attached to breakdown now impressed themselves on me.

By the time I was carried into the male admission ward of the Royal Dundee Liff Hospital I was expecting only the worst.

I looked around in horror. The walls of the dormitory were unpainted. Clumps of electric wire protruded from holes in the plaster. A few old, crumpled faces watched me as I was placed in bed. Seeing the partially redecorated ward my mind leapt to the worst conclusion. This was it. I had ended in the bottom of the pit. My first arrival in the bin.

As children we sometimes talked about going to, or more usually, being sent to the looney bin. The particular bin which featured in our games was Murthly outside Perth. My brothers would sometimes pretend to ring up Murthly to have them come and take me away. From such beginnings our preconceptions grow. But at that time I had never seen Murthly and had no idea what it or any other looney bin looked like. If I had been asked, I suppose I would have compared it to Perth prison. Nowadays, with the impact of television news and documentary features, public ignorance may be less rooted. Even so, there remains a common association of psychiatric hospitals with the Dickensian workhouse, and the output of the media has often hardened that impression. Eloquent pictures of long, bare corridors and large high-ceiling dormitories, or gaunt sprawling buildings overlooked by tall water towers, or laundry chimneys, confirm the feeling of a world apart, living on a different time scale. While hospitals such as these do exist, indeed it is not possible to conjure such pictures out of nothing, the reality that exists beyond the public image is a little different.

Variety is the main feature of the impressions I have acquired in the course of fifteen years in and out of bins in Scotland and England. It is true that the old Victorian and Edwardian mental institutions look remains at the core. Many outer suburbs of our great cities are dominated by these buildings. Epsom on the south-west fringes of London appears to be entirely encircled by them. But things are changing. The great expense of maintaining and improving the fabric of these old hospitals has given added impetus to the movement towards community-based care. New psychiatric units have appeared attached to general hospitals. Physically these could not be a stronger contrast to what went before. The first time I was admitted to one of these new units, I was quite uncomfortable with the hotel-like environment of decor and comfort. Not at all like the Spartan look to which I had been accustomed. Moreover, many of these units have superb equipment and facilities. But even among the old-style institutions there are variations. While some old hospitals vie for the dishonour of having the longest and gloomiest corridor in Europe, and others display workhouse architecture which is openly intimidating, there are others which in their way are magnificent. The Victorian predilection for siting asylums away from the urban centres in the fresh country air undoubtedly contained a large element of "out of sight out of mind". Even so, it did mean that these hospitals often have beautiful situations among fine and well-tended grounds. There is a N.H.S. hospital nearby to Perth which I almost deem it a privilege to have been a patient in, so elegant were its furnishings and decoration. It was the nearest I have ever come to living in a stately home.

13

Like many psychiatric hospitals, Royal Dundee Liff was a mixture of the old and new. My ward was part of a converted Victorian country house set apart from the main buildings. The main block was old, its passages haunted by long-term patients. On a rise behind the hospital there was a large O.T. department which was almost brand new and extremely well equipped. As so often, the hospital was set in its own grounds and surrounded by open countryside.

When I was more recovered, I would go walking among the fields or take a bus down to the centre of Dundee and have high tea on my own. But for most of the time the hospital ward was the centre of my life.

Psychiatric wards are highly individual. Each stay in a psychiatric hospital is flavoured by the fellow patients who share the time with you. There are significant differences too between an old-style ward and one organised on a therapeutic community model, between a segregated and a mixed admission ward. Nevertheless, this diversity hides a substantial similarity. The structures on which N.H.S. psychiatric care is built are remarkably uniform. The culture or subculture with which the mentally ill have clothed these structures is homogenous. The way of life, and the legends of life, which the mental patient acquires in hospital are similar across the country. At Royal Dundee Liff I first became aware of themes which were to reoccur unfailingly at all my subsequent admissions.

One of the most obvious differences between a ward of physical and a ward of psychiatric cases is that the psychiatric cases are not normally confined to bed. But if not confined to bed, they are quite often confined to the ward and its immediate environs. From this arises one of the most prominent characteristics of in-patient life for the mentally ill – creeping boredom. Boredom due to physical confinement in a hospital bed, boredom due to a legal confinement in a psychiatric ward, are burdens of their own. But boredom of the average mental patient is of a different nature. It is a peculiar oppression to be restricted to the sedentary life of day room and television room, not through compulsion but because the alternatives are less possible or less attractive. Thus, the hours of life on the ward are filled with idleness and the knowledge that everyone is waiting for something to happen. The deadness of these unfilled hours is the landscape against which all other hospital events occur. Psychiatric care is not a dynamic process. The inevitable boredom is compounded by the difficulty individuals often find in detecting any progress in their own recovery. Whereas in physical illness progress can be easily seen and confirmed, the symptoms of psychiatric recovery can be very gradual and the patient least able to detect it. The many hours spent in hospital chairs become tinged with a combination of boredom, helplessness and frustration. At Royal Dundee Liff, I saw my relationship to time change. The hours and their significance expanded while my powers and significance shrank. It is claimed that rest is a great healer and I have no doubt that it plays an often-uncredited part in the restoration of mental health. Even so, the inertia which hangs shroud-like over many individuals in the wards and rooms of psychiatric hospitals is a weight it is difficult to accept.

Within this inertia, waiting is a dominant component and within the category of waiting, waiting for doctors plays a prominent part. At Royal Dundee Liff, we were always waiting for something to happen – waiting for the next meal, waiting for night-time medication, waiting for health to overtake us. But among all these, waiting for doctors was the most significant. It absorbed most time, consumed most energy, gave rise to the greatest frustrations. One of the most elemental rules of psychiatric life is the unavailability of psychiatrists. Almost by definition the psychiatrist is harassed and overworked, an expert whose time is at once extremely valuable and carefully apportioned. It almost seems that a psychiatrist who is not very busy is a psychiatrist who has lost his self-esteem. At any rate it should soon be apparent to the patient that he must not expect to see his psychiatrist too often. I have from time to time wondered how many minutes patients do spend with psychiatrists during the course of an average admission and whether these justify the high position the psychiatrist maintains in the hierarchy of carers. Certainly, such time must make up only a very small percentage of the patients' total time in treatment. It quickly becomes apparent that it is an advantage to accept you will see your doctor when he asks for you rather than vice versa. In this way, you spare yourself much wasted expectation and benefit from occasional welcome surprises. The processes of mental hospital have a slow and steady beat. Unfortunately, too many of them seem to be experienced from a recumbent position in an armchair.

Alongside the boredom and waiting mentioned above, and arising in some part from them, is another easily detected characteristic of ward life – hostility towards doctors. I have experienced a definite underlying resentment, on my own and others' part, that people should be expected to reveal all about their private lives to strange doctors. The idea that remote emotionless doctors can cut your ulcers out is easier to accept than that remote emotionless doctors can tell you how to run your life. While we normally accept the expert's position in relation to medical problems, this position is more precarious when it comes to psychiatric areas. The feeling: "Who the hell does he think he is to tell me how to ...." often hovers unspoken in the atmosphere of the day room. As a consequence, the unbridged rift between the interests of the doctors and the patients is seldom completely obscured. After all, we have become through illness broken down human beings and must resent, however covertly, others who claim they can restore us to our full humanity. It is less easy to accept advice than a Band-Aid.

But as a corollary to these tensions is the presumed right to medication. While many patients may resent analysis of their life from a psychiatrist of a different culture and origin, they will often accept a dose of drugs from the same person. Large numbers of patients, in my experience, feel that they should be medicated while within a psychiatric ward. Indeed, they feel they have a right to be so treated. They may feel they are not being treated properly, or at all, if they do not receive some form of medication. In general, patients tend to assume that psychiatry, like all other forms of medicine, is the arena of physical treatments. This balance of expectations when taken in conjunction with the balance of therapies normally offered may do something to explain the inert character of much ward life. This was very much my perception when I first encountered psychiatric hospital life at Royal Dundee Liff in the late 1960s. I still believe it is an important element in the 1980s. There has been change. Ideas of psychology and the dynamics of so-called relationships are now an integral part of much media output. Supportive groups, self-help groups and agencies covering problems of all kinds have blossomed. The barriers against talk-oriented therapies have been weakened. At the same time the drugs revolution in psychiatry has run its course and been replaced by a general awareness that chemotherapy is not the simple panacea many had been led to expect. Today the incoming psychiatric patient may have a more flexible expectation than many had in the 1960s and 1970s. Even so, the underlying reluctance to discuss the secrets of your life with a doctor and a persistent hope that simply swallowing tablets can solve everything remains an important strand in the backdrop of ward life today.

Royal Dundee Liff was my first taste of the bin, and I learned a good deal from it which was incidental to the progress of my treatment. It was my first real taste of an adult world and to a large extent it was an alien world. I remember watching epileptic fits, holding down a man with D.T.'s from potato-wine. I remember standing to attention by our beds when the consultant did his round and how he would cross question us like army recruits in front of other patients. There was also much laughter and kindness from fellow-patients amidst the atmosphere of an emotional climate where the patient was still an isolated individual and looked to the experts rather than his neighbours for real help. I did not, in particular, acquire a sense of resentment from this first period in hospital nor on this occasion a defined self-image of myself as a mentally ill person. The lessons I learned did have a longer-term effect. Nevertheless, in the immediate sense it was how little Royal Dundee Liff changed me which was to be of greatest importance.

1.02

CAMBRIDGE – THE GOLDEN LAND

I did recover at Royal Dundee Liff. By Christmas I was ready for discharge back to the community and what I expected would be a normal life. There are many reasons for recovery from a breakdown. Among them a cloistered life, at least three meals a day and plenty of opportunities for sleep may not be the least significant. But amongst those which are more commonly acknowledged, consultation with a psychiatrist and medication were paramount in my case. The powers of chemotherapy cannot be gainsaid. Regardless of its impact on the real problems, chemotherapy has a most observable effect on symptoms. My acute anxiety was controlled and the subsequent lethargy and depression balanced largely through the medium of oral medication. My psychiatrist, in contrast, merely sold me a rather loose and diluted Freudian interpretation of my life and times. This seemed, on the one hand, irrelevant and, on the other, made my relationships with my family a great deal more difficult. I suppose it is unfair to expect psychiatrists always to get it right at the first attempt and, at this time, they were working without the benefit of a convincing diagnosis of my case. Nevertheless, it was from this instance that I developed a suspicion of attempts to insinuate a free-floating interpretation of life onto the patient-victim. To understand and accept an expert's analysis of your life and situation may have inherent benefits. Everyone is looking out for meaning. But unless this explanation converts itself directly to action in the present and the future its value must be limited. Too often understanding, in a psychiatric context, is an undeveloped potential. Too often the chance for action in the real world is never realised. Many psychiatrists seem to read out the words and then exit left, leaving you on the nursery floor to make the best of it. I do not believe we should allow psychiatry to be a religion and practise on N.H.S. premises at the same time.

In the main area of personal change, my psychiatrists at Royal Dundee Liff were unable to succeed. My determination to return to Cambridge for the following year survived unshaken. Unfortunately, in their attempts to persuade me against this, the staff chose to attack my strongest unit – my academic ability. Instead of emphasising the social and emotional problems I would encounter, they chose to suggest that I was not academically or intellectually equipped for Cambridge University. This I refused to accept. With some justification, in view of the fact that I had won a minor

DOI: 10.4324/9781003636434-5

scholarship to study there in the first place. My intellectual ability, proved in the open market, was the one thing I was convinced of and would not surrender lightly. The more pressure was applied, the more resolute I became. In the end the valid arguments that were introduced simply failed to make any impact. Thus it was that I left Royal Dundee Liff with my sights set on return to Jesus College the following October. In no major respect was I better equipped to deal with the problems university life would again pose except that I was, to some extent, forewarned by the previous autumn's events. I think I felt things would work out somehow, and I think perhaps the psychiatrists were too kind to disillusion me.

I did not leave hospital scarred by the months I had spent inside. I did not feel I was marked out from the rest. I viewed my breakdown as some still unexplained hiatus in my normality and did not feel affected to any greater extent than if I had suffered a severe physical illness which had now cleared up. To bog your breeks once may be an accident, not significant in itself. But in some ways, I was changed. I had done a fair amount of reading while in hospital – books about mental illness and psychology in the main. This information, combined with my everyday memories of ward life, began to alter my outlook on life. Social conscience, which my education had not notably developed, now began to assume a larger role in my thoughts. To some extent, I had been on the lower rungs. I certainly felt that I had been there, and looked on this as something extra, something special for one my age. The negative aspects had not yet been revealed. The difference which a spell in the bin had brought was not a separation. I felt more of an individual but still within the body of my contemporaries. If I felt myself marked out from my peers at all, it was for a vaguely positive quality rather than for any shameful stigma.

The months following my discharge seemed to confirm that I had stepped back easily into normal life. While waiting to return to Cambridge I took two jobs, one in a ski-hotel in Glenshee near home, the other as an assistant to the warden of a youth hostel in Shrewsbury. At Glenshee, I was part of a close-knit staff team forced by the isolation of the hotel to rely on each other's company, while in Shrewsbury I was isolated in the middle of a city with a warden who for some reason completely ignored me and hardly ever spoke. Both situations taught me a great deal, in particular the fact that I survived my first real encounter with loneliness while at Shrewsbury made me feel that I had enough strength to return to my studies and be successful. For six months I had been living in the real world, away from home, beyond the protection of Royal Dundee Liff. I felt I would be starting on a completely fresh page when I got back to college. I cannot remember even being particularly worried at the prospect.

I had arranged to return to Jesus College for the Long Vacation term in the summer, before the academic year began in earnest in October. This spell in Cambridge, without the pressure of lectures and studies, passed off successfully and I felt prepared for the real test. It is possible that I was over-confident. It is possible that most of the problems which had triggered my original breakdown had not been confronted at all. Whatever the reason, when the academic year did begin, I only just made it.

Whereas the previous year I had reacted like a scalded rabbit, this time I became manic. At any rate, that is what I choose to call it with the benefit of hindsight. I did not lose contact with reality in the sense that I believed I was someone, or something, else or that I was unaware of my actual surroundings. But my connection with reality was modified. Instead of withdrawing in shock from a reality which appeared overwhelming as I had done before, I now attempted subconsciously to accommodate that reality through my own modification of it. Instead of holding the truth external, and saying that I could not fit into it, I denied various aspects, and in some areas replaced them with my own more acceptable version. I suppose this may be a more sophisticated way of dealing with unpleasant difficulties. Certainly, it was a more complicated response than my blind panic of the previous autumn. But perhaps because it did not focus on my own self-separation from the environment, my new strategy enabled me to stagger through the first weeks of term. But only just. Because my behaviour expressed itself in manic ways, in other words because I was over-active, excitable, aggressive, there was no doubt that I seemed strange to many people in the college, including the establishment. I did not endear myself to my first supervisor when I declared I would write all my essay assignments in verse rather than prose. In the end, my parents came down from Scotland again, and through them I was warned that if I couldn't shape up, I would have to drop out. That message penetrated. Somehow, I managed to pull myself together sufficiently to satisfy the college authorities.

The overflowing of the dream into real life is a symptom of madness according to the poet Gerard de Nerval. Bernstein, a pioneer of modern psychiatry, remarked that "in truth we are all potentially or actually hallucinating people during the greatest part of our lives". In fact, the complex relationship between fantasy and reality in our everyday life should be more broadly accepted, if only to underline the direct path that leads from so-called normality through neurosis to psychosis and beyond. Although it is possible to speak of someone, of oneself, losing all contact with reality, the vast hinterland which lies between such a boundary and the equally far-flung territory of complete contact with reality is the more important area of concern. It is here that most people make their own accommodation to the acceptable or unacceptable faces of their life. It is here that people choose for the long term or short term to adopt degrees of unreality into their makeup. This is a common process and may not be remarkable. It is when it becomes evident in unusual behaviour that it becomes significant. Behaviour is one of the main foundations upon which psychiatric diagnoses are established. Certain behaviour by patients in mental hospitals is taken to be evidence of schizophrenia or of manic-depressive psychosis, depression or anxiety neurosis. Different behaviour defines different diagnoses. In a similar way, in society as a whole behaviour is a benchmark which helps decide whether you are mentally ill or normal, sane or mad. The man who said that, if you must go mad do it discreetly, was a man of wisdom. Thus, it is possible to believe that the High Street is full of green elephants, or that you are John Wayne, and yet live outside a psychiatric unit, providing you don't talk to too many people about it, and refrain from acting as an elephant hunter, or riding shotgun on the Corporation buses. During those weeks of my first term at Cambridge, I survived because I was just able to restrain my behaviour within the boundaries acceptable to that place and time.

In a sense I was fortunate that I was a student in a Cambridge college. Provided I did not act outrageously, and produced one piece of written work each week, there were minimal demands made upon me. Had I been called to work a nine-to-five, five-day week, or operate in close conjunction with other people, I should probably have disintegrated completely. As it was, my eccentricity was tolerated. I stumbled through the first term. During the last two days before I returned home for Christmas, I had a period of violently unpleasant delusions, during which I lost all contact with place and time. It was the first time I had really experienced madness and was, in many ways, a foretaste of future episodes. Nevertheless, on this occasion I returned spontaneously and outwardly undamaged. For the next eighteen months, until the completion of the first part of my degree, I was to all intents and purposes an ordinary Cambridge undergraduate.

It is not easy to write truthfully of my years at Cambridge. I look back now on those days with much bad feeling. But at the time I would not have wished to be anywhere else. Cambridge had been my promised land as a teenager. In a sense it was to remain so for a number of years. Having won a place to study there, it took me five years and three breakdowns to gain my degree. During that time, I never seriously questioned its value and importance. If I look back, and consider my Cambridge days as a bleak, bleak time, it is because my priorities now are not what they were then. In retrospect, Cambridge defined what I was not, and separated me from my peers and from the expectations we had held in common. Yet, at the time, I was happy for long periods and, almost always, convinced of my ultimate success.

I did not return to Cambridge as an outsider. My stay at Royal Dundee Liff had not left me handicapped in that way. Nevertheless, the incidents during those first weeks of term were the beginning of a process which was to move me to the fringe of college society and eventually to the position of an outsider. I became aware of having acted strangely within the college and was ashamed. This forced me in upon myself, a position I was to retain and perfect during the subsequent years of my student life. Allied to my suspicion that my contemporaries thought I was odd, was the simple truth that Cambridge University life didn't suit me very well. College society seemed to be divided up into a warren of little groups and societies, membership of which was essential to convivial functioning. To sit in hall for evening meal in the middle of one of those groups without being an acknowledged member was like auditioning for the role of the Invisible Man. Having started on the wrong foot, my obstinacy made it essential that I balanced on that foot for long periods. I can remember going for periods of five or more days without speaking to anyone in those early days. The sense of living an unreal life in an unreal environment stays firmly in my mind even now. In the end I found my niche among the small group in my year whose main characteristic was that they had no obvious niche. Throughout my five years at Cambridge all the friendships I did make were with undergraduates who themselves had few friends. The social life, the activities which make up the popular image of the Cambridge experience, completely passed me by. Academic life was my priority. The demands of college society and my own natural inclinations, with very little aid from the pressure of ex-mental patient status, were already dictating that my social posture would at the least be that of the loner.

The late 1960s and early 1970s were special years at Cambridge. It was a time of much student unrest. The Vietnam War had stimulated concerned protest from young people throughout the western industrialised nations. This was amplified in Cambridge, and in other universities, by protests over the running of faculties and by internal disputes about programmes of study. Everywhere students were campaigning for more control of their courses. This period was that of the Greek Colonels regime. In Cambridge protest against this regime led to the so-called Garden House Hotel riot, resulting in the trial and imprisonment of a group of students. It was a period of change, attempted change and controversy.

Although I did not become politically active in the usual sense, the prevalent atmosphere did influence me. I felt that much political work in the university still revolved around the clubs and the debating chamber and that the realities of life in the city of Cambridge went largely unnoticed by many students. As a result, I worked with the Cambridge Simon Community or, as it was to become, the Cambridge Cyrenians. This group works to provide care and support for the homeless and rootless, the dosser or the vagrant alcoholic. Throughout my time in Cambridge, I worked extensively for the Cyrenians and they became the focus of my non-academic activities while at Jesus College. Apart from social conscience, the main stimulus for my involvement was the experience I had gained while in psychiatric hospital. I identified consciously with the dosser's position. The work was an act of defiance against my own family and society as a whole. The pressures of living in an environment from which I had fled a year previously, and into which I was not able to readapt, moved me towards a more concrete definition of myself than had proved necessary in the months immediately after my discharge from Royal Dundee Liff. I was more conscious of being rejected. I was now identifying myself with the have-nots rather than the haves. However important the genuine elements in my motivation were, however much I may have achieved in real terms for the Cambridge dossers, my work with them was a significant element in my own search for a comfortable identity.

Nevertheless, there was a large element of romance in this. The role of outsider, its pride, defiance and tragedy, is attractive. My cultivation of the role was still, at this time, due more to a generalised perception than to a true feeling that I was separate, or separated, on account of one mental breakdown and three months in a looney bin. There had been some valid incidents which could help justify a self-image of the upper-middle class boy made bad. But, in truth, I did not feel that there were real barriers placed between me and my contemporaries because of my previous mental status. Nor did I, and this was of equal importance, have a significantly different outlook on life or markedly different goals. We were still on shared territory. At this point, I neither wished nor was I being pressured to stand outside the boundaries of my immediate society. Although I did not operate easily in the system, for a year and a half I operated within it, concentrating on my studies, intent on success in that area. In the broadest terms, the progress of my career was moving satisfactorily.

In the summer of 1970, I was awarded a first in History and a scholarship for my final year's study. This result I took as no small triumph. It seemed that I had confounded the judgement of the psychiatrists at Royal Dundee Liff and this gave me a double satisfaction. But, in the main, I was delighted that hard work had gained reward. For two years, my studies had been my main concern and enjoyment and the examination results confirmed that, whatever my shortcomings in other areas, in the field of academic endeavour my value was considerable. I still clearly remember driving down from our farm to the nearest town to read the results in *The Times* and feeling somehow changed by the success announced in its pages. It seemed like an affirmation and a breakthrough. I was in the swim again.

In fact, this achievement was a prelude to greater disaster. During the summer vacation I returned to Cambridge to prepare a fund-raising campaign for the Cyrene Community. I lived in their day shelter in a disused Cambridge public house. Shortly after my arrival, the community leader went on holiday. While he was away, the deputy-leader was dismissed and I, as the only person available who knew the dossers, took control. The stress was too great. Very quickly, I became hyperactive and eventually broke down in the West End of London while on my way back to Scotland for a rest. My eldest brother rescued me in the early hours of the morning in Soho. I had been wandering the area with a dog called Moses convinced that there had been a nuclear attack and that we were the only survivors on the surface. I was a long way out this time, well into the territories of looney behaviour. After a brief, and nightmarish, few days in St Bernard's Hospital, Southall, pacing the ward incessantly, and making feeble attempts to escape, I was transferred back to Scotland under escort. I remember approaching the Highlands in the evening and noticing that the old lady opposite us on the train had a Campbell tartan bag. I took it as a sign. Whether it was of a homecoming, or the old closed circle, or both, I don't think I was certain.

My destination was Murray Royal Hospital on the edges of Perth. Murray Royal was an extraordinary place. As different from Royal Dundee Liff as Dundee, an old industrial city, is from Perth, a sedate county town. In terms of appearance, Murray Royal is the most remarkable bin I have ever stayed inside. The exceptional comfort of the wards, the furniture and fittings, and the care with which they were maintained, reminded me more of a stately home than an N.H.S. hospital. I am sure memory has played me false to some degree. Nevertheless, I have largely pleasant memories of Murray Royal. After my initial crisis had subsided, it was not a time of torment for me. In a large part, this was due to the fact that I was in the care of an exceptional consultant. The nature of the psychiatrist's job often seems to make it difficult for him to act like a normal human being. At Murray Royal I was fortunate. Among the psychiatrists who have treated me, this gentleman, the only one that I have believed, was consistently concerned about me as an individual. He was the only consultant who was courteous enough to fulfil promised interviews even if it meant coming on to the ward at eight o'clock in the evening, and the only psychiatrist I have known who would send apologies through the staff if for any reason he could not be present at the hospital on a day he was due to speak with me. Whether or not his prescribed treatments changed my life, under his care I was treated as a feeling person. In the context of present provisions, I believe his concern was exceptional. He is the only psychiatrist I have met in the last eighteen years that I would accord unreserved respect.

I was an in-patient at Murray Royal for the best part of six months. At Christmas 1970, I was discharged but my father died suddenly over the holiday period and that precipitated my early readmission. When I finally left hospital, my goal, as before was to return to Jesus College and my final year. In the hope that I might return and complete my studies, the college authorities had once again given me a year's leave of absence. My determination was still to beat the challenge. But things had changed. One breakdown is very different from two breakdowns. A large part of the confidence I had acquired after my examination success in June 1970 had dissipated by the time Easter 1971 came around. In June 1970, I had believed myself in the mainstream. By Easter 1971, I could see that was a fiction. I pretty much knew that the breakdowns were not simply going to go away. My psychiatrist had diagnosed me as a manic-depressive, a diagnosis which all my subsequent consultants were to follow. While this was progress in a sense, and there is a perverse comfort in having a secure diagnosis, it did saddle me with the prospect of being, as it were, mentally ill for a continuous period into the future. Whereas my first breakdown had left me with only an indistinct feeling that something was permanently amiss, by the time I left Murray Royal this perception was tangible. My separation was becoming crystallised. Moreover, my father's death marked the end of something. The family sold up the farms, and my mother moved down to England. From 1971, my home-land was no longer my home. Although I did not realise it at the time, a true end had been marked. In some ways, I never addressed myself to the idea of return to my academic studies. In a sense, I would merely be going through the motions. My determination to finish what I had begun overruled the truer instincts of my heart.

My final year at Cambridge developed into disaster almost immediately. During the course of it, I discovered that a number of my supervisors had been surprised to see me return at all. They clearly felt that an honourable retreat would have been more understandable. This was the first time that I began to consider my per-sistence might actually be self-destructive rather than the only acceptable course. Unfortunately, by then things had gone too far. Almost immediately the autumn term had begun, I became manic and disappeared into the centre of London over one weekend, experiencing delusions, fantasies and strange ideas. Suffice it to say here that I was a missing person for a few days, that I ended up incoherent in a padded cell at Banstead Hospital, South West London, saying only that I was Peter and that I came from Jesus. Within six weeks I was back at college, still hoping to sit my final examinations the following June. Now I remember Banstead chiefly for two reasons. The first its intimidating workhouse architecture, the second that it was while there that I first underwent electric convulsive therapy.

The speed with which an individual may cross into and return from madness is remarkable. I am able to pass from recognisable normality into missed contact with reality, and thence through terror and despair back into functional normality again, in the space of ten days or less. Clearly, modern mood-changing drugs can control such episodes and facilitate speedy return. Clearly, there are many whose journeys are more profound, and whose return from such destinations may never be total. Nevertheless, my own experience, mirrored by other written accounts, is that spontaneous journeys into, and out of, madness over relatively short periods of time can, and do, take place. This should be a salutary reminder that the boundaries of madness, let alone its true nature, are not coherently defined. We should not relax ourselves into easy preconceptions of the cataclysmic nature of such phenomena.

I still had an outside chance of making up lost time and gaining a degree. But, in truth, my admission to Banstead had put paid to my hopes. My confidence was shattered and, more vitally, my concentration effectively destroyed. Over the next couple of months, I was increasingly undermined by the realisation that I was disintegrating as a competent individual, let alone as a third year History undergraduate. At last, halfway through January 1972, I was admitted to Fulbourn Hospital, outside Cambridge, with depression. There I was to sit out the remaining months of my degree course, satisfy the residential qualifications, and hopefully qualify for a special aegrotat degree. It is the only time I have ever been admitted on the grounds of depression.

My entry into Fulbourn effectively ended my five-year courtship with Cambridge University. During those years my fixed ambition had been to achieve a good academic success. As long as this remained possible, and clearly my judgement of possibilities was not always very concise, my determination had been to continue. Through continuing I retained, in my own assessment, a position in the mainstream of my contemporaries. My goals and their goals were similar. While the chance remained that I too would fulfil those goals, then my links to my peers were preserved. By the summer of 1972, this construction of my internal and external worlds could no longer hold. Mental illness – for such it was commonly described – had prevented me from achieving my clearest goal. It was no longer possible for me to feel part of the same commonwealth as my peers. I was separated from society, both my immediate society and its wider equivalent. Although I was granted a special aegrotat degree, I felt I had failed. Already I could say that mental illness had changed my life.

In June 1972, I was awarded a B.A. in History and left Fulbourn Hospital. In many ways I learnt more at Fulbourn than at any psychiatric unit before or since. Fulbourn was certainly the most imaginative hospital environment I have experienced. This reaction may be partly due to the fact that while an in-patient in Fulbourn I was never in a situation of crisis and thus better able to benefit from the facilities available. Nevertheless, I do consider Fulbourn as one of the all-too-few places where I have seen mental health tackled in a creative way. Even so, my developing career as a psychiatric in-patient was not interrupted markedly by my stay there. Within three months of leaving Fulbourn, I was admitted to West Park Hospital Epsom. I was to remain an in-patient there for almost exactly one year.

1.03

BREAKDOWNS AND SHAKEDOWNS

Half-way down Elgin Avenue, West London, a quarter after midnight and my stomach went. For two days I had been aware of going high. Now I knew I wasn't going to be able to hold on by myself. Eyes half-closed, talking to myself…. Head down to the pavement to cut out the senses. Got to make it home. Stop remembering the other times and that irresistible urge to run off into the darkness. To lose myself.

I lie in the bed-sit. Everything is feeding me. Carpet, cups, walls, all accelerating my thoughts. I know I'm going to run out into the streets. No buses. No tubes. Hours till daylight. I dial 999. Very calmly, I explain that I'm a manic depressive and I'm having a panic attack. The listener is totally unimpressed. Clearly this is not his idea of an emergency. I sit on the stairs and wait. Five minutes later he returns and says that my duty general practitioner (G.P.) will call me back.

I make tea and wait. Tidying. Anything to keep me in that tiny room until the phone rings. After ten minutes the G.P. calls. He is also unimpressed. He doesn't know me and clearly has no intention of making my acquaintance in the foreseeable future. He offers a prescription. I ask for someone to talk to. No chance. Mate.

Thank you for your degrees and qualifications doctor and your telephone number. I'm off to Middlesex Hospital Casualty Department and you can tell them I'm coming if you want. My anger and frustration force me back into reality. I should have learnt from experience by now. When you're really in trouble, go to the source yourself. No messing.

This time I was lucky. I had six pounds 50 pence in my wallet and a taxicab was coming down Abbey Road as I ran out of the house. Next time I'll try saying I've cut my wrists and see what happens.

Mental breakdown is not an act of God. Despite its unexpectedness, its traumatic consequences, breakdown is a phenomenon which can be approached on a practical and rational level. It is important to re-assert that the individual can work towards control of his breakdown process. Even more so, the principle is that he should be given the chance to attempt this. Mental breakdown is a classic declaration of loss of control, a public statement of the separation which underpins the mental patient's negative status. If the individual patient, or ex-patient, is to recover his full status the experience and process of breakdown must be returned within his domain.

DOI: 10.4324/9781003636434-6

I believe the importance of the breakdown experience in mental illness cannot be overemphasised. My own experience as a manic-depressive is, I admit, particular. It may well be unusual to have more than ten admissions over a period of fifteen years. This may have made breakdowns especially significant to me. My own history is individual and may not be characteristic of manic depressives as a whole, let alone of other diagnoses. Moreover, it is undeniable that the majority of people who suffer mental distress receive treatment from their G.P.s and are never admitted to a psychiatric unit at all. Thus, the full-blown breakdowns that I have experienced, leading to a period as in-patient in a psychiatric hospital, may only affect a small statistical minority among those with mental health problems. While I accept all this, the experiences of those with whom I have shared hospital wards since 1967 are not insignificant. For a period of years, I have worked to win control of my breakdown process – to move from uncontrolled disintegration to a controlled and limited relapse – and there are many I have met who have struggled towards the same goal. In some respects, this must be seen as a goal separate from the broader changes we seek in our lifestyle. However much I may change the quality of my life, my status, my grasp on happiness, I can never escape the memory of severe breakdown. The fear that something may go wrong and that I, in breakdown, may destroy myself remains, however prolonged my grasp on normality has been. To modify the destructiveness of the next relapse is a specific, and separate, aim which may bring its own substantial security. It is an aim akin to damage limitation. In this sense alone, if in no other, the importance of the actual process of breakdown remains central to the lives of all mental patients, present or past.

Breakdown and admission into psychiatric care is the first and most important foundation of the labelling process which accompanies the so-called mentally ill as they progress through life. In a sense, breakdown and admission remain the clearest, and most popular, indication that an individual is mentally ill and thus separated from the normal majority. These events mark a demonstrable crossing of the line. Their importance in the broadest sense is highlighted by the fact that recovery and discharge from psychiatric care is not taken as implying a crossing of the line in an opposite direction. To this extent, breakdown is always a one-way journey. It is a transition which cannot be reversed.

The disruptive effects of breakdown are significant on a number of levels. Not only is the personal, internal life of the individual overthrown, but his relationships with immediate friends and family are altered. Furthermore, breakdown has an impact on a wider stage. Admission involves administrative and bureaucratic procedures which mark out a change of status. Alteration of position is formalised in Department of Health and Social Security records, tax records and employment records. The individual's descent to mental-patient status seems to be indelibly recorded for the future purposes of society. In reality, this may not be a true impression. But it is often how it can seem for the victim. Moreover, the wide-ranging repercussions of a breakdown cannot be denied. Only the fortunate emerge from breakdown and admission without losing either housing or employment or both. Dislocation occurs on microscopic and macroscopic levels.

Symbolically, and in practical terms, the process of breakdown has a central significance for the mental patient.

In the face of this traumatic event, and of the need to subject it to some degree of effective control, how much assistance does the prospective mental patient actually receive from existing facilities? A simple answer might be – not very much. In my experience it is often extremely difficult to gain the kind of help one wants in times of crisis. Indeed, there is sometimes a feeling that the person in breakdown cannot, by definition, be in a position to properly know what help he wants. In general terms, National Health Service (N.H.S.) psychiatric provisions are not attuned to provide a sensitive response to breakdown. The philosophy behind such responses as are available often seems openly inimical to the idea that a victim can extend personal control over his predicament. The belief that a breakdown is a breakdown and not part of a continuing life-process seems to motivate many psychiatric responses to in-patient admission. The possibility that people might actually wish, and need, to remain involved in the process of their breakdown is not often entertained in any practical way. Obviously, admission procedures occur at the sharp end of hospitalisation. Many in-coming patients are distressed – frequently they may be resisting admission, or objecting to their treatment, in disruptive ways. While this is happening, nursing staff will often be expected to carry out the many bureaucratic formalities which seem necessary in such transitions. Thus, both the incoming patient and the welcoming staff are placed under considerable strain. Even so, the consideration given to the real needs of the patient at this time may not always be a priority, let alone the thought that he or she might have some insight into what those needs might be.

One of the factors influencing the new admission's state of mind is the ease or difficulty with which he has been able to secure assistance in time of crisis. There are many ways of ending in the bin. If you take an overdose and are brought into hospital on a stretcher, then I believe the emergency services are competent. If you do strange things in the street, or climb monuments in the nude, then the police service is more than adequate. But in the wide area between such extremes, an area where the individual may wish to retain some involvement in his own fate, the picture is more varied. Both in terms of choice, and in terms of flexibility, the facilities have important limitations.

The General Practitioner is the hub of the National Health Service. He is a natural first destination for people in mental distress. Often, he will, of his own resources, be able to deal in some measure with the mental health problems presented to him. If not, he will refer patients to other specialist agencies – psychiatrists, psychologists, counsellors. On occasion, he may himself be instrumental in effecting the speedy admission of a patient into a psychiatric unit. Throughout, the G.P. remains a key figure in the system, so that any recourse to assistance that bypasses him may prove fruitless. It is, for example, not rewarding for an individual in crisis to present himself at a psychiatric hospital, or admissions unit, asking for help directly. The normal form is to proceed via the G.P.

Such a system has limitations and I shall discuss the role of the G.P. in more detail in a later section. Obviously, effectiveness depends to no little extent upon the level of psychiatric knowledge prevalent among G.P.s, the relationship between the G.P. and his patient, and the frequency of their contact. There may be times when one, or all, of these elements are missing. It has been my own experience, over a period of frequent changes of address in North West London, that the poor communication between G.P. and psychiatrist, coupled with an absence of common information, made coherent care impossible. The strain involved in having two experts with such divergent approaches, and uneven information on my case history, involved in my care was such that many years ago I made the decision to keep my physical and psychological complaints entirely separate, and to avoid ever involving one expert in the sphere of the other. Commuting from one decision to another was simply too exhausting and expensive. This decision was a voluntary and individual choice and may well have been eccentric. Nevertheless, it is an indication of the type of problems which exist in a system so dependent upon the proper functioning of the G.P.

But there are situations where recourse to the G.P. is not appropriate. Emergencies are one of such situations. If you feel that you are losing control, that you need immediate help, in particular if this becomes apparent during the hours of darkness, one of the few sources of help that may be open is the casualty department of a general hospital. My own crises have frequently developed with great speed. On a number of occasions, I have found myself alone at 1:30 in the morning contemplating my own disintegration and wondering where to turn. It is at these moments that one realises the paucity of alternatives. For this reason, I would not wish to be overly critical of the facilities casualty departments provide. If there were more suitable destinations, if G.P.s responded to calls with visits rather than on the phone prescriptions, people like myself would not have to seek out casualty departments and take pot luck. Often the treatment dispensed there is sensitive, and more than adequate to meet immediate need. But I have been turned away from a casualty department when clearly in need of treatment. Once I was sent packing when suffering the severe side effects of a phenothiazine drug and collapsed in the street half an hour later. I have often felt that to arrive at a casualty department, and complain that you are having a breakdown, is to invite the staff to treat you as though you are mad. Casualty staff are not trained to be experts in psychiatric care. It is not reasonable to expect them always to be fully conversant with psychiatric treatments. I have found staff who knew less about psychotropic drugs than I do. Casualty departments are available. They provide a welcome place of safety in a time of crisis when no other asylum is clearly to be seen. They provide a service across the whole range of medicine and their shortcomings for specific psychiatric needs are because they were not designed for such needs, and because there is nothing else that is. They are a resort, but anyone who travels to a casualty department in the expectation that his psychiatric needs will be met travels with false hopes.

It may seem unjustified to stress such problems. After all, I am not complaining of neglect or active mistreatment. Besides, everyone is aware of the frustrations involved in obtaining help through the N.H.S. While I accept this to be true, and in no way question the dedication of those who man the front lines of N.H.S. care, I do not feel this precludes protest. This is doubly so because the effects on the psychiatric consumer are likely to be heightened. If I ring up a psychiatric hospital where I have previously been an in-patient, and where my current consultant works, and am told that I cannot see her even though I believe I am approaching a crisis, what kind of response is this in human terms? If despite this, and the knowledge that I am going counter to procedures, I consider my position so serious that I travel 30 miles across London to that hospital and am then kept waiting for six hours even though the consultant is in the building, how much of my agitation is due to illness and how much to being treated like a naughty boy who has broken the rules? If the stress of obtaining treatment actually increases the symptoms of illness for which treatment is sought, then this should be recognised and the problem confronted on the victim's behalf. It is ironic, that I, as a veteran of numerous admissions, should be intimidated in times of crisis not only by the memories of previous illnesses but of the battles that I have undergone to receive proper treatment for them. The desire to avoid another trip through the grinder may be an unhighlighted reason why many ex-patients deny their illnesses and avoid recourse to professional help until beyond the vital moment.

Throughout the practical problems of breakdown and admission, there is one important element of conflict – the conflict between achieving the help you want and being given the help someone else, usually an appointed expert, thinks you need. Wants and needs are seldom reconciled in psychiatry. Conflict between psychiatrist and patient is a hallmark of mental health. The cult of the expert has been under increasing attack in contemporary society. The accepted wisdoms of physical medicine are now challenged by alternative medicine, herbalists, allergists and many more. But in psychiatry it is more doubtful that there have ever been accepted wisdoms in a real sense. Professor Szasz has spoken of psychiatry as being the field of competing visions and philosophies, more like an area of beliefs than of science. Certainly, there seems to be a much wider divergence of interests between experts and consumers in psychiatry than elsewhere in medicine. Goals and methods are openly challenged or resentfully endured. It might even be claimed that the relationship between doctor and patient in psychiatry is based on opposition not co-operation. At present, I wish to emphasise that conflict between carer and cared for is a dominant aspect of psychiatric life and that it is during breakdown and admission that it often finds its most forceful expression.

My own belief is that the process of breakdown can be controlled. In my view, an individual may reach a position where he can anticipate the onset of crisis, retain some control over it and, even if driven to seek admission into a psychiatric unit, remain in charge of himself with the cooperation and support of the trained staff available there. This does not seem to me to be an outrageous thesis. Nor should it be considered as something more than the so-called mentally ill should expect. I have already outlined some of the practical difficulties the individual may confront in obtaining his needs through the N.H.S. Of equal significance are the philosophic obstacles which surround the individual as he negotiates breakdown.

It often appears that the experts do not wish the individual to remain in control during a breakdown. It is certainly not a priority during admission. If remaining in control implies that the individual has some opportunity to express opinions regarding his immediate treatment and needs, in particular if such opinions contradict the professionally controlled process, then such control is often discouraged or manipulated away. During breakdown and admission, as in other phases of life on the ward, the impression that a good patient is a submissive one is hard to avoid. These attitudes, however damaging to a patient's short-term or long-term integrity, are not consciously malicious. In my opinion, they spring directly from procedural convenience and the belief that the patient is somehow incapacitated beyond cogent involvement as a result of being in the throes of breakdown. Such an approach seems to me to be supported by two ideas common among National Health staff and confirmed to some extent by the literature. The first is that breakdown is somehow separate to the individual experiencing it. The second is that many people in breakdown, particularly those with certain diagnoses, have no insight into their condition.

My manic depression when it is under control seems to be a part of my total being. When it is not completely in my control, so that I must seek professional assistance, my manic depression is treated as a disease, a virulent bug, an outbreak of symptoms which must be acted upon with scant recognition of its relation to me, a living, developing human being. In a sense, manic depression is treated no differently from malaria. While dormant, malaria is viewed as a potential within the blood. Once it erupts again, the response is to take emergency physical measures to control and suppress the eruption. The re-emergence of mania or depression is often treated as an outbreak of disease distinct in itself, connected more with previous breakdowns than with intervening periods of health and self-development. Hospital staff often react to the event and not the life.

To some extent it is inevitable that breakdown and admission should be seen as a peculiar event, separated from the less traumatic stages of in-patient treatment. There is a certain validity in the assertion that people in acute distress cannot come to terms with the true problems underneath their symptoms. Perhaps this may help explain the easy resort to medication at times of admission. Nevertheless, not all breakdowns are the same. They must be differentiated. By treating breakdown as a separate event, by isolating it from the full life-history of the patient, the danger arises that degrees of breakdown will not be recognised. The patient becomes the victim of the professional knee-jerk. The manic patient can only have a manic relapse, the schizophrenic a schizophrenic one. The framework of previous years becomes the prison of future behaviour.

In breakdown, it is common for the victim to disagree with the treatment which is being chosen for him. There may be many reasons for such objections, some of them valid some invalid. Unfortunately, the possibility of deciding the validity of any objections is somewhat prejudiced by the widespread belief that many of the mentally ill have no insight into their condition and that this is particularly true in times of crisis. The concept of insight is a fascinating one for anyone with mental health problems. In the wrong hands, it could probably write-off two-thirds of the population of the United Kingdom. Many years ago, when I was a teenager in a Scottish psychiatric hospital, I remember a very sympathetic charge nurse comforting me by saying, "You'll be alright son. You've got insight". At the time I felt some divine blessing had been conferred on me and was encouraged. Since then, my experience suggests that a substantial number of professionals believe in this supernaturally bestowed insight, a quality you either have or have not, and which cannot, almost by definition, be acquired or developed. It is commonplace to read that a characteristic of schizophrenia or manic-depressive crises is a lack of insight. Yet I have met many schizophrenic and manic-depressive patients who were fighting like tigers to retain their integrity during crisis. It is not uncommon to hear certain individuals dismissed largely because an expert has allocated them a particular diagnostic label after they have shared their company for less than two hours over a period of three months. If having insight is merely another species of labelling, then it should be thrown out forthwith. If lack of insight is simply another way of denying an individual's point of view, prejudging options during break-down and admission so that the expert's course of action is always pursued, then it is both a tool of oppression and an incentive to shoddy nursing practice. Insight must be viewed as a dynamic possibility. If we cannot learn, then what is the point of psychiatry? But, at the same time, the possibility of insight must be recognised across the spectrum. It is no good to recognise insight in a placated patient in the Day Room and deny its existence in a disturbed new admission. It is not necessarily true that a schizophrenic patient with no insight during one breakdown must be a schizophrenic patient with no insight during the next one. While it may be less convenient to recognise this and to act upon it, only by doing so can the humanity of the breakdown victim be respected.

To illustrate the above criticisms, I would like to cite two separate admissions I went through a number of years ago. These two episodes involved the same hospital, the same consultant psychiatrist, the same admission ward and a number of the same nursing staff. I had been associated with the hospital for some years. I had been having regular manic relapses at eighteen-month intervals and I was well-known in the hospital. The first time a relative drove me to hospital, I was agitated but, after some discussion, agreed to be admitted. I was given a large dose of chlorpromazine and sent home to collect some gear. When I returned, I was given another large dose of chlorpromazine and the formalities of admission were begun. Half-way through these, while being interviewed by a junior nurse, I lost consciousness. Three or four hours later, I awoke and the admission procedures were completed by the evening staff.

Some years later, I arrived at the same ward and asked for help. I was asked to remain as an in-patient. I was upset and reluctant but did not oppose this. While waiting for the duty doctor, I stayed on the ward and talked with some of the patients I knew from previous visits. When the doctor came, I agreed to take some medication and we talked for ten minutes about the differences between the English and Indian education systems. I was perfectly coherent and the doctor seemed unconcerned. I was then given a liquid dose of chlorpromazine. Within a few minutes, I was staggering around the ward, completely out of it, and eventually had to be put to bed by a male nurse.

Such unfeeling, and undifferentiated, drugging out illustrates the worst side of the admission process. On neither occasion was I a threat to myself or to others; indeed, on the second occasion I left hospital after ten days and have not since returned. Nevertheless, the automatic reaction was not to talk to me, or give me any coherent attention, beyond routine questions about personal property and sickness benefit forms, but rather to drug me into unconsciousness. I still remember those two admissions as a gross insult to my human rights. Many ex-mental patients speak of their treatment in hospital as punishment. I do not adopt this view. But instances, such as those above, confirm to me the mindless lack of caring which the present system tolerates. After fifteen years work to win control of mania, I do not take lightly casual drugging out which destroys in me another chance to successfully negotiate it in my own way. If I felt saying "Hands Off" would make matters better, I would repeat it throughout each new admission. In the past I have been out of control. I have been admitted in such states that medication alone would control. But should I, and others like me, always be victims of our past behaviour, should our agitation always be ascribed to psychoses susceptible only to medication, should we be automatically denied the chance to master the crises which dominate our fears? Sometimes, it seems, once a nutter always a nutter, is the only available choice.

To protect the individual's right to participate in his predicament, it is perhaps necessary to look for alternative systems to those commonly provided by the N.H.S. Any journey whose destination is of necessity the psychiatric admission ward is a journey – to separation and powerlessness. The social and institutional realities dictate this. The victim expects that his arrival in a psychiatric hospital marks the crossing of a line, a separation from the active self-controlled life of society. The necessities of bureaucracy and professional care merely confirm this to him. By entering the present system, he surrenders himself into the hands of others. His inabilities are emphasised and broadcast. Indeed, to some extent they become essential to his successful sojourn within those asylum boundaries. In short, the transition which breakdown represents is everywhere distorted and perverted by the environment in which it is forced to occur. Breakdown can then only be seen as clinical, destructive and anti-life, a nightmare from which nothing of value can be gleaned.

But it is not always inevitable that a psychiatric hospital should be the destination. In recent years the value of crisis intervention services which aim to keep individuals within the community has been recognised. In reality, there are extremely few such crisis schemes, and I have no experience of them, or of anyone who has used them. The choice open to people in breakdown remains inadequate. Indeed, the interests of diplomacy are the only thing that could argue for the use of the term choice at all. While alternatives do exist, while alternative philosophies recognising the need for flexible and unstructured responses to breakdown continue to win support, the pattern of care upon which most must rely reacts with only grudging movements to the patient's need to be a participant in, and not a victim of, their own life process.

In the end, the assertions I have made in this chapter must be founded on my own personal experience. In eighteen years of dealing with N.H.S. psychiatric provisions, it is events which occurred during the phase of admission to hospital that I remember with the greatest resentment. I have already indicated that such a phase is, perhaps, the most difficult for all parties, and to some extent this may explain my reaction. Even so, it is my impression that insufficient attention is given to the best treatment for individuals during breakdown. Too often the simplest and most convenient response is the one chosen. Irrational behaviour, which is after all not the prerogative of people in breakdown, seems to encourage the belief that the patient is not aware of what is going on and will not remember arbitrary treatment, particularly if it brings his unstable and destabilising behaviour to a swift end. Nothing could be further from the truth. Many ex-mental patients are keenly aware of the dehumanising implications of their status in society's eyes. We are, therefore, more than sensitive to unnecessary reductions in our integrity which professional carers inflict during admission.

In all this it is important to ask whose best interests are being served by current procedures. I still feel my progress towards control of my life has often been hindered rather than helped by professional responses. Rapid recourse to drugging out is not always the key to self-knowledge. It is significant to me, as an experienced practitioner of the mental breakdown, that no-one in all the N.H.S. hospitals I have frequented has ever given me advice on how to manage a breakdown once it has begun. This is the professional's job. The victim should lie back and let it happen. It is only when he has emerged through the tunnel, when his driving licence has, as it were, been endorsed and his self-image carefully squashed, that rehabilitation can begin again. The mental patient's position will only significantly improve when professional expertise fully accepts our rights even during breakdown, and treats the process of breakdown as a vital part of a continuing life story, and not a caesura and an aberration.

1.04

LIFE ON THE INSIDE

I am an admission ward person. I am not a back ward person or a locked ward person. Nor am I an alcoholic ward person or a therapeutic community in a hospital ward setting person. I have on occasion been locked up in padded cells and I have some experience of life on a locked ward. But in the main my time in the bin has not been spent under lock and key and what knowledge I may have of life on back wards is confined to casual observation, and to a period helping in one, while I was an in-patient on an admission ward. Thus, my views on life inside the bin are from a particular perspective. I do not claim a comprehensive vision. On the other hand, I believe much of what I have experienced in admission wards has a wider relevance and is shared by many others among the population of psychiatric in-patients.

In the 1980s, one is more likely to spend numerous short spells inside the bin than one long stretch. This is one of the major changes in the experience of mental illness over the last 50 years. To be diagnosed as the victim of a mental illness which needs treatment will not now commonly result in one being separated from the society of one's contemporaries for periods of years or even decades. Nowadays, more people are likely to find themselves popping in and out of the admission ward once or twice every three years than languishing in a back ward. A recent Greater London Council (GLC) survey of mental health in the London area showed that in only one borough in the GLC area were fewer than 50% of admissions discharged within a month. At the same time the survey showed that the ratio of readmissions to new admissions was in the order of 3 to 1. Whatever else these figures reveal, and their implications are important, they confirm the nature of the psychiatric patient's current experience. Short stays on admission wards, frequently repeated and interspersed with periods in the ordinary community, do not conjoin to produce the same attitudes and expectations as fifteen years in a long stay ward. One of the major problems in contemporary psychiatry is that professional attitudes to mental illness have not always moved as rapidly as the attitudes of the so-called victims. Too often, the inhabitant of the admission ward is expected to behave as though he were institutionalised, without having the necessary track record on which to base such a performance.

DOI: 10.4324/9781003636434-7

A major feature of the admission ward environment is that it is volatile. The admission ward is frequently described as an "acute" ward. The exact meaning of the word acute in a psychiatric context may not be clear. But one aspect may well mean "not under control". The behaviour of people in admission wards is "not under control" in two contrasting ways. You are quite likely to find fellow patients acting in unusual ways. Individuals may repeatedly lie on the floor in crucifix positions. Others may take their clothes off during "News at Ten" and expose themselves to the newscaster. People may talk openly of the devil, sorcery and witchcraft. These, and other unexpected behaviours, may not be commonplace. Nevertheless, they do occur and can prevent the atmosphere of the admission ward from attaining ordered calm. On the other hand, the environment is also "not under control" because many new admissions are extremely upset, and their quite natural agitation has not yet been brought within the influence of mood altering medication. Thus anger, fear and confusion, – perfectly reasonable reactions to the stresses involved in breakdown and admission – tend to survive in the admission ward. The volatility of admission ward life is not merely due to the fact that some patients display blatantly unusual and disturbing behaviour but because a much larger number are displaying perfectly appropriate signs of their distress, and that this has not yet been modified, as it might have been in a long-stay psychiatric ward.

I do not believe physical violence is a characteristic of the admission ward. In a way it is rather surprising that it should not be so. Most people who decided to pack their front room with angry and aggrieved people would probably expect some of the china to get broken. I have only been attacked twice in eighteen years as a user. Both times by the same patient within the space of two days. I have certainly seen some incidents of physical violence between patients – on one occasion resulting in serious injury. Yet I do not consider admission wards are violent in that sense of the word. In the same way, I have witnessed incidents where violence was inflicted on a patient by a member of staff. Such cases are inexcusable, but as far as I know they are exceptional. Most violence on admission wards is directed at the self and not at others.

Hostility is a different matter. There are many reasons why a patient has hostile feelings associated with his so-called illness and those who treat him for it. Social attitudes to the subject of madness and the physical and psychological processes involved in psychiatric care are prominent among those which come instantly to mind. Whatever the reason, the anger that admission ward patients feel about their own predicament, coupled with resentment against professionals who claim they are providing treatment, is an enduring element in ward life. Nor should it be assumed that hostility is only one way. In my experience, many staff are covertly hostile towards in-patients and, in some cases, their underlying hostility may find expression openly both in words and in actions. It is not unknown for staff who will call you a "barmpot" or a "nutter" to your face to continue in National Health Service employment with the backing of their colleagues. If the admission ward is not a stage for regular outrage or violence, neither is it a model of the extended family playing pass the parcel after Sunday lunch.

There are several more mundane reasons for the admission ward's volatility. One is the mixture of people that will often be found there. The first admission wards I stayed on were single-sex wards. More recently they have always been mixed wards and I believe that this is the popular trend. Combining men and women within the same ward may seem to be a natural development and to have numerous advantages. It can also bring its own problems – as the number of complaints of sexual harassment alone will testify. Of equal importance is the fact that admission wards contain a very broad range of diagnoses. The inclusion within one ward of patients who may be acutely depressed, acutely agitated, acutely alcoholic or acutely geriatric creates obvious strains. With the current understaffing of psychiatric wards, these problems are exaggerated. I have been in admission wards where in order to care properly for two or three psycho-geriatric patients, an understrength nursing team has had to ignore the rest of those on the ward for the greater part of both morning and afternoon shifts. It is not difficult to imagine the atmosphere of a closed environment where people who are acutely depressed, immobile and uninvolved are mixing with people who are extremely agitated, hyperactive and interreacting. When such a mixture is being supervised by an understrength caring team, which is itself struggling to cope, nobody should be surprised that words like turbulent and volatile can sometimes be used in descriptions. Indeed, what is remarkable is the overwhelming tolerance displayed by all parties to the situation, and in particular the in-patients, who are after all supposed to be malfunctioning in one way or another in the first instance.

Things change quickly on admission wards in some respects. I remember occasions when I have been admitted to a ward that was dominated by depressed and psycho-geriatric patients. Within a week four other "manic" types have arrived and the ward has been turned upside down in all senses of the word. Manic-depressives may not rule the world, but a couple can run most admission wards no bother. I've seen a patients' kitchen transformed from a haven of calm to a refreshments factory capable of producing a hundred cups of tea an hour, and delivering tea and biscuits complete with tray and doilies to every new arrival in the ward, patient or staff, within three and a half minutes. Not only that but we fertilised the entire Day Room and Television room with tea leaves at no charge whatsoever. On long-term wards it is more likely that a sleepy atmosphere will remain a sleepy atmosphere for months. On an admission ward the emotional climate may revolve in a complete cycle every month or five weeks. In this respect it is a special environment within an environment.

I do not wish to describe in detail the everyday routine of ward life. I have already described some of its characteristics in Chapter 1.01. Psychiatric wards have always reminded me of public schools with some of the same stratifications of society and intricate games playing. As in the public school, there is an upper strata of doctors or teachers who are in control of the show but are, in actual fact, isolated from their patients or pupils, and have little or no insight into the special myths and culture of the people they are caring for. Helping the doctors are nurses, much like prefects in their closer contact with the ordinary inmate, their devoted

administration of numerous, often nonsensical, rules and regulations and their ultimate insignificance in relation to the power and status of their superiors. At the bottom of the pile are the beneficiaries of the system, playing and winning their own
little games, swearing in the toilets, getting drunk on weekend leave or stepping on
the quadrangle grass when no one is looking.

In fact, there are numerous games played in admission wards. Often, they
are played with an enthusiasm on all sides which betrays the vacuousness of the
underlying, and artificially constructed, environment. Sometimes they are merely
endured or actively resented. One of the most prevailing games that I have encountered is the "Let's get the patients to play games" game. This is an effective and
much practised strategy which is irritating without carrying the obnoxious implications inherent in other heavier games. It seems to be based on the belief that a
person is somehow better off if he is pushing a set of draughts about, playing gin
rummy or, best of all, playing Scrabble. My experience leads me to suspect that
some psychiatric nurses are addicted to draughts and Scrabble. Indeed, it may well
be an inherent predisposition among the nursing profession as a whole. I do know
nurses who could clear the Day Room in three minutes by closing the medication
trolley and declaring "Anyone for Scrabble?". I have also taken part in the longest
game of Scrabble in National Health Service history. This lasted for four and a half
days. Someone actually began the game, was discharged, readmitted and back at
the table on the final evening to complete the closing moves. I am quite an accom-
plished Scrabble player, but I have on occasion dreaded the after supper press-gang
which emerges from the nurses' office. Sometimes resorting to table games reflects
a nurse's loss of imagination, not a patient's need for distraction.

A more portentous game altogether is the "we are observing you" game. Observation is an essential element of psychiatric care, particularly as diagnosis and
treatment depends so much on observed behaviour. This fact need not lead to
oppression. But it does mean that patients are aware of being watched and that a
gentle paranoia underlies their day-to-day activities on the ward. For example, it
is very common for new patients when presented with a boiled egg and a plastic
fork to suspect that their response is being tested out, rather than that the student
nurse is short-sighted. Incidents like this become common currency of Day Room
conversations. In the same way, the staff's insistence on always putting the record
player and amplifiers in the quiet room may well be viewed as a Machiavellian
design to uncover psychosis.

In reality, direct observation is a fact of life and must be tolerated or subverted.
Nursing staff have to learn, to report back to senior nurses and doctors and this
often involves the in-patient in bouts of being stared at. The most annoying and
persistent form of observation I have encountered is the "observation at mealtimes"
sub-group. I am not keen on eating in large public places, particularly hospital caf-
eterias. To be half-way through a plate of porridge at eight in the morning and discover your escort nurse sitting three tables away peering at you like an ingenuous
heron is guaranteed to kill your appetite. Of course, nurses must do what they are
instructed to, and they are not permitted to eat with patients, but their obtrusiveness

still offends me. The only groups of nurses I have ever known to be effectively surreptitious in the meal-time observation game are those from Malaysia or Hong Kong. The only effective response to this type of surveillance in my experience is either to complete the eating process in less than five minutes, or to sit directly opposite your observer at the same table and stare it out.

Not far behind "mealtime observation" in frequency and often surpassing it in absurdity is "student-allocated observation". This occurs when a student nurse is allocated one or more particular patients as subjects of study. Shortly after he has been so allocated the individual will be confronted by a student nurse, perhaps one to whom he has not previously spoken, who will corner him in a chair and ply him with questions: "What diagnosis do you think you are?" "What month is it?" "Do you think your manic-depression is due to studying too hard for your A Levels?". I am not averse to answering questions about myself. Indeed, the demands of the psychiatric process can turn you into quite a performer. But I do find the charade absurd and demeaning. Is it impossible for the student nurse, or the charge nurse, to approach me openly concerning this study? Why the secrecy, the play-acting? Why the assumption that I cannot tell the difference between a normal conversation and a grilling about my "case"? The answer is a mystery to me. Perhaps professionals think we would all tell lies if we knew what was going on and that we will not if we only suspect we are being pumped. Perhaps they fear we would tell them to get lost if they gave us an open choice. Perhaps they would rather we carried the paranoia as well as them.

Absurd as these things may appear to the outsider, they are not insignificant. The nursing staff and the in-patients are the two largest elements in the community of the admission ward. Divisions enough exist. They do not need to be widened. Moreover, there is a danger that the nurse will acquire attitudes which allow them to treat in-patients as specimens or objects of study, and separated from them, rather than as ordinary human beings. I do not believe this is an idle fear. I was once in another admission ward to my own at a birthday party. I was sitting on the floor. Most of the chairs were taken. A student nurse whom I had never seen before and who was not involved in any way in my care approached and began questioning me as to why I was sitting on the floor. I replied that I wanted to. This did not satisfy him, and he proceeded to harass and cross-examine me for some minutes with questions, many and varied, including "Who is your doctor?" "Do you know why you are here?" "Do you know what a chair, a table, is for?" – followed by his own explanation. "Why won't you sit on a chair?" and so on. In the end I left the party, to which I had been specifically invited, and returned to my own ward. This incident is extraordinary in many ways, but it is an event which occurs somewhat more than seldom in psychiatric institutions. Questions from a question master may elicit precious information. They can also turn the supplier into a victim and the questioner into a tyrant. On admission wards the line between benevolent acquisition of information and exploitation is finely drawn. Too often the standard practices encourage the belief that the in-patient stands in a degraded relationship to those who orchestrate his care.

One of the strategies which would seem to contradict the patient's diminished status is the provision of ward meetings involving the caring team – doctors, social workers and nursing staff – and the patients. At these occasions, matters of importance to the life of the ward are discussed. The antecedents of such ward meetings are not entirely clear to me, and I am sure they vary from hospital to hospital and from area to area. Nevertheless, I can claim that none of those with which I have come in contact, or which others have described to me, seem to have much connection with the therapeutic community ideals of Maxwell Jones. That Maxwell Jones was a pioneer in social psychiatry is not open to doubt. What is less clear is how much practical effect his ideas have had on the general shape of psychiatric units in the National Health Service. It is a source of much regret and anger to me that many professionals seem so proud of token innovations like weekly ward meetings and do so little to introduce the substance of Maxwell Jones' approach. It really is a case of praise Maxwell Jones and pass the hypodermic.

The reality of those ward meetings in which I have participated is that they are limited in scope and entirely dominated and controlled by staff presence. Although a patient may take the minutes, the chairman is always a doctor or social worker controlling who may speak and for how long. It is not uncommon for someone to be cut short when entering awkward or upsetting subjects and the whole meeting to be brought to a close because the social worker has another appointment – regardless of the importance of the subject under discussion at the time. In general, the concentration on washing-up rotas, cleanliness and complaints about diet merely highlights the power of the staff and the powerlessness of the patients. At the same time, co-operation among patients in problem solving is not stimulated. Recourse to the experts is confirmed and extended.

In all this, what is worrying is not only the poverty of the ward meeting as a device but the satisfaction most of the caring team display regarding its function. The ward meeting does not to my mind in any way meet the need of the individual to be involved in the environment, human and physical, in which he is being given treatment. The hierarchies of power are merely crystallised and demonstrated to him through his attendance at such meetings. The message he receives is this – Do the washing up. Make your bed. Otherwise leave it all to us. The ward meeting enables the staff to salve their consciences. It does nothing for the in-patient. The powerlessness which is the dominant condition of the admission ward dweller is merely deepened.

This is the crux of life on the inside, the context within which everything else occurs. For in the admission ward the powers of the patient over his own life are rather small while the powers of the professional worker over the patient's life are rather great. This is evidenced not only by the fact that if someone decides you need a large injection of a tranquilising drug, and you disagree, there is little in the final analysis that you can do to avoid it, but also in more subtle and insidious ways. The patient is certainly not in control and attempts to regain control may be viewed with great hostility and suspicion. Of course, power may be exercised benevolently and often it is. Nevertheless, the whole area of mental illness itself is concerned with power and loss of power, of loss of self-control and resumption of self-control. This complicates the argument considerably. Thus, while on one level the professional's assumption of power within the psychiatric ward may be necessary, benevolent and guided by the long-term interests of the patient as far as they are perceived, on another the patient's exclusion from power can do nothing but heighten his degradation and confirm the feeling of self-worthlessness which his breakdown has already engendered. Separation from power is also separation from health.

Some years ago, and a few weeks after discharging myself from hospital, I returned to my former ward and spoke with one of the charge nurses. During the conversation he said I would no longer be welcomed in his ward should I ever return. Both he and his staff, or so he claimed, objected to me being admitted and then complaining about the treatment I received and the fact that my consultant would not speak with me. I find the implications of this incident disturbing. How much of it was occasioned by the fact that I had gone against the expert's opinion, discharged myself, and was surviving (and incidentally have continued to survive), I cannot really judge. But what it does suggest is that compliance is the price of care to certain psychiatric professionals. As long as I was compliant and co-operative, I was welcomed. As soon as I asserted my own demands, and made complaints about the service provided, I was threatened with refusal of future treatment. I have never attempted to subvert the authority of nurses or doctors on admission wards. I have never advised fellow patients not to take their medication nor attempted to persuade them to go against their doctors' advice. Throughout my periods on the admission ward over which the above charge nurse had authority, I spent a deal of time helping and supporting staff and patients. On the one occasion, when I was involved in a formal complaint against a staff member I did so with great reluctance, and only because I was directly asked to do so by a senior nursing officer. In short, it was hardly my revolutionary posture which was provoking such a reaction from the charge nurse. It seems more likely that this particular incident may have arisen because I actually felt – rightly, as it transpired, that the treatment I was receiving, and the environment in which it was taking place, was inappropriate, and spoke out over it. The underlying assumption that the experts are doing you a favour for which you should be grateful was thus challenged and the nurse's sense of injury resulted. If these attitudes of "Doctor knows best" and "you can like it or get out" actually lurk behind the professional facade of the expensively trained charge nurse, then I think the average in-patient can understand why the atmosphere sometimes makes him feel uncommonly prickly. Surely it cannot be inevitable that transactions between patients and the caring team should be so tightly circumscribed, that the patient must be slapped down if he calls the nature of the process into question?

Staff on admission wards are notoriously sensitive to criticism and will reject even constructive suggestions if they contain hints of adverse comment regarding their role. Their rules and their own identities are of understandable importance to workers in a psychiatric environment. Separation between the caring and the cared-for is to some extent inevitable. Nevertheless, it is depressing how often when the crunch comes, the staff will choose to maintain their own corporate identity and the distance between themselves and the other major group sharing their environment. Co-operation in a psychiatric ward is predominantly a one-way affair.

On one occasion, I was at a weekly ward meeting where the patients were being criticised for leaving the kitchen untidy and were told that it would be locked up except at certain times. In our defence we pointed out that we made tea for the staff when they came on duty morning and afternoon. This was no palliative. In a further attempt to point out that we did try to help ward staff, I reminded them that I had for well over a week been looking after a severely depressed woman – helping her down to the cafeteria, making her eat. This too was no palliative. Indeed, rather the opposite. "You have no business interfering with other patients. What if she fell down? What would our union say?" came the reply. Strangely enough, the conversation ended there, and the meeting immediately after that. It is at times like these on an admission ward that you realise that whatever category of human being the in-patient comes into, it is certainly different.

Attitudes like these, whether due to professional self-regard or the absence of some other quality, limit the potential of the admission ward. Perhaps it is necessary that its potential should be limited but the result is that the experience becomes alien and the individual who is at the centre of the experience becomes sooner or later alienated by it. I would find all this more excusable if the system worked. I might be happy to be hit over the head six times a day with a blunt mallet if it proved to be an effective way to become a bright eyed and successful member of society. But the system is demonstrably not working. The ratio of readmissions to admissions I cited earlier in this chapter shows this. The psychiatrist, the psychologist, the therapist and the nurse do not have access to a superior and inarguable wisdom. It is quite wrong for them to carry on as if they did. Very often they may have less practical understanding of what they are doing than those they are trained to help. It seems absurd to me that there is so little interchange between the members of a psychiatric community, that hierarchies are established which close off real communication, and prevent most intelligent attempts to discover just exactly what is going on in this process called mental illness.

I believe that patients on admission wards should be treated as equals and not as prisoners in someone else's world picture. The paralysing nature of mental illness is not solely due to biochemical malfunction. Nor yet to the bio-chemical juggling which is the most common response to it. It is also due to the attitudes displayed to patients while they are in psychiatric wards. For, whether consciously or unconsciously, the caring team in its function regularly makes the in-patient feel that there is something wrong with him as a human being, that they cannot allow the patient, for some reason, to be "all there" while on the admission ward and that his interactions both with his fellow patients and with them must remain limited, unfulfilled and something less than the normal citizen would expect.

My intention is not to paint the psychiatric in-patient as an innocent cast into a forest of monsters. Many people who go through the admission ward are cared for in their distress and emerge profoundly grateful to the staff. Life on the inside has constraints and a large number of these are unavoidable. But some can certainly be avoided. The resentment many ex-patients feel must come from somewhere. It is not a precondition of mental distress. Nor do I believe it is sufficient to call on the "peculiar nature of the phenomenon of mental illness" – potent though it may be – as a blanket alibi. It may possibly be that the admission ward is not the perfectly designed environment. Personally, I have no doubt that the conditions on admission wards, the presence there of people who should have been better cared for elsewhere, the inability of professionals to deal humanely with those who end up in the system, provides a particularly fruitful breeding ground for negative feelings. Like it or not, many psychiatric patients feel trapped and punished. Whatever else life on the inside may impress upon you, it prepares you for the likelihood that from hereon in, you are likely to be well out of the mainstream, son.

This is a particular quality of life on the inside: that it is a reflection of life on the outside. The pricking kindnesses of the nurses, the dismissive care of the psychiatrists, are subtler aspects of the blatant prejudgements which take place in the wider community. Professionals may act as a focus, but they are not the true source of light. However much I may resent the ethos of admission ward caring, I must sit in the Day Room and admit that it is at least caring, and that beyond in the society to which I aspire things in general are much worse. That is where the feeling of being a secret society springs from, that is why manic depressives sit in the television room in the middle evening to pun and make limericks and spin in-joke tales the nursing staff cannot absorb. That is why, when I hear them complaining about it in the ward office over their coffee cups, I feel good. At least we've got a few punches in before we go out to our own pummelling. To some extent, life on the inside always has the feeling of a trap within a trap.

It is not real life on the inside. Its nature depends on the existence of a real life on the outside. Essentially, to live on the inside is always to be a presence in an absence, to exist removed from existence, to be a non-entity. I have not met many in-patients who did not want to return to the mainstream. However scared we might be, we know the difference between stork and butter. We didn't choose to go inside to make some brave political statement. We are caught in a limbo, and we are quite aware of it. The worst times I have ever had were when I lost belief that I could go back and live on the outside. That was when so-called mental illness came closest to destroying me. Not the times when I was manic and dreaming of the Martians.

There is a special time in psychiatric wards. It is the witching hour: The hour between the arrival of the night staff and the distribution of night-time medication at ten o'clock. At this time, with only one or two nurses on the ward, with night coming on, people tend to gather in little groups and talk in a different way. These are the minutes when I have felt most strongly what it is to be mentally ill and on the inside. It is at this time that the implications of our predicament tend to be discussed, and that the strength of madness in all its senses is most acutely realised. Sometimes I have felt that we were all touched. It is too easy to dismiss such ideas as romantic. One of the major problems in this area of concern is that people want to confine it to a peck of powder in the bottom of the jar. If we spent more time thinking about the night and less about processing symptoms of illness through standardised mechanisms, perhaps life on the inside would feel less like a plate of oat flakes and more like a decent meal.

THERAPEUTICA – CHINKS
IN THE ARMOUR

My year in West Park hospital Epsom included a full range of in-patient experiences. I was admitted onto an open ward but became so distressed, and my
behaviour so uncontrollable, that I was moved to a locked ward. There I ended
in a padded cell refusing to eat. I remember very well lying semi-naked on a
mattress in a bare room. I remember spending much time with my eye squeezed
to the spy-hole to see if there were any humans on the outside. I remember too
almost dislocating my neck trying to batter my way out. Sometimes the door
would open, and a group of nursing staff would look in on me. It is not safe to
assume that people do not remember significant amounts of what happens to
them when they are quite disturbed. I remember, indeed I cannot forget, a great
deal.

Eventually, I was allowed into the body of the locked ward, and sometime later
back to my original ward, the unlocked admission ward. There I improved, or did
not improve, over a period of some months during which a variety of drug therapies
were tried out and I was pressurised into undergoing a series of electric shock treatments. Finally, it was agreed that I was recovering suitably under a particular drug
treatment, this was stabilised, and thought was given to what should happen next. I
seemed to have emerged satisfactorily through whatever it was I had been assumed
to be going through at the outset.

For the last four months of my year in West Park, I was marking time. Although
my mood was stabilised under drug treatment, my consultant was unwilling to
allow my direct return to the wider community. Instead, a place was sought for me
in a therapeutic community, a half-way staging post, as it were, between complete
dependence and complete independence. Meanwhile, I kicked my heels and waited
for the chance to move out.

One of the major weaknesses of the old-style mental hospitals that I have experienced, indeed I believe it is a weakness of the system as a whole, is the inadequacy of facilities for those approaching discharge. Individuals who have regained
a certain degree of health but are not yet deemed ready to return to normal life often
find themselves marooned in some species of limbo. On this particular occasion,
the length of my being delayed from discharge was probably exceptional, and the

DOI: 10.4324/9781003636434-8

reason for my delay based on a true perception of my long-term needs. Nevertheless, it did reveal the poverty of resources available to someone in my position at that time.

Although I was not thought to be ready for return to the community, neither was I in any way able to benefit from the hospital facilities which were offered to me. The caring team didn't appear to know quite what to do with me. At a certain stage, I was moved away from standard occupational therapy, perhaps because something more directed was considered necessary, perhaps because the experts wished to anticipate my boredom. Instead, I was transferred to industrial therapy on the pretext that it would prepare me more effectively for real work. The "real work" industrial therapy actually offered involved sitting at a desk for hours assembling plastic World War II tanks or filling little tea bags with teaspoonfuls of mixed herbs. Needless to say, this was agonisingly dull work and dispiriting in the extreme. It did not nicely meet my needs as I perceived them nor bear much relevance to the type of employment which I, as a recent graduate, still hoped myself capable of achieving. In general terms, I find it difficult to see that "real work" of such a kind has anything but marginal value. In retrospect, it seems to say much for the valuation of many in-patients that they had and, I believe, still have to, endure such debilitating and soulless work without choice and for a few pence an hour.

I eventually graduated from industrial therapy to what was known as I.T.O., a form of industrial training. This training took place in a grubby workshop outside the hospital in Epsom itself, and involved me in long hours soldering leads or cutting sheets of plastic and polythene. In some ways I.T.O. was the top of the ladder as far as working opportunities at West Park were concerned. The fact that it related in only the haziest sense to any of my real needs and expectations of employment was in retrospect probably irrelevant. I believe the priority was to keep me occupied, not to equip me in any serious way for the demands of employment in the real world. My hands were not idle. I was kept busy and off the ward – indeed outside the hospital entirely – for large portions of each weekday. In terms of what was then on offer to most at West Park, the industrial therapy and training opportunities made available to me were probably generous. Nevertheless, I did little more than vegetate for four months. I was contained within a form of custodial care. I was not stimulated or drawn out of myself in any way. The psychiatric system was quite prepared to treat me. But to educate or change was quite another matter.

So it was with a combination of much relief and intense apprehension that I finally heard that my place in the therapeutic community had come up. As the autumn began, I left West Park and headed for North Kensington in London. I had never lived in London before. I had no friends in London. In reality, outside of one or two people I had met inside the bin, I had no friends period. I remember being shown through the slightly dishevelled building off Ladbroke Grove which housed the community and being left with my baggage in the bedroom I was to share with another resident. I remember wondering casually what it must be like to jump out of a first-floor window. I felt lost.

One of the main purposes of a therapeutic community, as I understand it, is to use to the maximum benefit the therapeutic capabilities of all members of that community whether they are staff or residents. The resources of those who are seeking help are recognized and valued as an important contribution to the potential of the environment in which they are living. In this way alone a therapeutic community will tend to differ from a hospital ward community. Vertical access to hierarchies of increasingly expert carers is off-set or complemented by horizontal access to the support of fellow community members. As the community becomes more truly a community, its capacity to be caring increases. That is one powerful motivating ideal.

Certainly the community in North Kensington differed in major ways from hospital. There were no doctors or consulting rooms. There were no nursing staff wheeling in trolleys of medication, no chivvying to stand in line for high tea, no roll calls or curfews. These and other absences, regardless of the underlying ideological approach, made a significant difference. To sleep in a fifteen-bed dormitory which is attended each day by a cleaner, a job protected by the union, is one thing. To share a small, badly furnished room in a grotty house for whose cleaning you are yourself partly responsible is something else. Sometimes it is a relief to know you are not supporting a vast service industry. Sometimes unpolished linoleum breeds a lesser paranoia.

The members of the community were also different in certain important respects from those I had encountered in psychiatric wards. The staff team were not in general trained in a medical approach to mental health problems and were certainly open to a much wider range of techniques than was common in psychiatric units at that time. It is perhaps not without significance that the only friendships I have ever made, and maintained, with staff involved in my care were established with members of the team who worked in this community. The emotional climate between worker and client was fundamentally different. The residents themselves did not necessarily come from a psychiatric background. Although a majority had been in psychiatric hospital and some, like myself, came directly from in-patient care, there were some who had been in only peripheral contact with psychiatry. Moreover, and most significantly, the community members were not usually in acute crisis when they entered the house. Unlike an admission ward which is constantly taking in people who are blatantly distressed, either because they cannot cope with day-to-day life or because somebody is telling them this is the case, the people who joined the house in North Kensington were, on the surface at least, more in control of their lives. They were more likely to be those thought to be coming out from under rather than those going down for the third time. As a result, although there was often a high degree of emotional distress within the community – indeed the nature of the community often encouraged more expressed emotion than might usually be found in a hospital – this was of a different character and expressed in different ways than in the crises of an admission ward. For this and other reasons the community provided a more stable base from which to tackle our problems.

Each of us had one of the staff as an individual counsellor with whom we met for a formal session usually once a week. The whole community met together once a week for a meeting which was partly business and partly discussion of general and personal issues which involved the entire house. Immediately afterwards we split up into small groups with five or six residents and two staff where personal issues were discussed more intensively. It was also a feature of community life that anyone in crisis could call an emergency house meeting to which everyone in the building at the time was expected to come. This range of group meetings was novel to me with my experience of standard admission ward practice and it certainly allowed a substantially greater involvement, a healthier intercommunication. It did not entirely resolve the problem of power sharing between carer and cared for. Conflict between residents and staff remained a theme of life in the house. Indeed, because staff were so much more approachable, so much more personally available within the community, conflicts were if anything more intense and more passionate. But at least differences were more open and more honestly expressed. The remoteness of psychiatric staff, and the facade of professionalism that submerges so much opposition into unexpressed resentment, was fortunately absent.

Ultimately power did reside with staff. Although residents were involved in many decision-making processes, being a necessary part of the selection group interviewing new applicants, for example, when there were major disagreements on important issues, the staff view would usually prevail. On one or two occasions there were violent incidents between residents. This was against the house rules. I remember arguing strongly against the staff position that the offenders must leave, not so much because I opposed the destructive implications of violence in a tightly knit community, but out of solidarity with fellow-residents and against the power-bloc of the staff. Nevertheless, the common areas of contact, communication, shared work, and shared leisure which the community life allowed quite overbalanced the inevitable tensions between the two groups. Compared to West Park Hospital, and what had gone before, it was another world.

By the time I reached the therapeutic community in Autumn 1973, I was at a crucial stage. I was already well launched into my career as a mental patient. I had spent a year in West Park Hospital. Since the summer of 1970 I had spent 25 months in one psychiatric unit or another. It was becoming increasingly difficult for me to decide just what my natural environment was. Although I was not yet institutionalised in the common sense of that term, my outlook on life was significantly coloured by concepts of illness. Months of separation from the real community while at West Park Hospital, months spent playing skittles against other psychiatric hospitals in South-East England and returning home in the hospital bus, months wondering whether it was feasible to live beyond the hospital gatehouse, had sown seeds of self-doubt. I was beginning to think in terms of what might have been instead of what could still be. By the time I entered the Richmond Fellowship house, there was a good chance that I would become a well-practised "patient", defending myself within the boundaries of that role and trapped on the magnetic inner circuit of hospital, day hospital and hostel. I was already thinking of myself as a case of manic depression first and as a competent adult second. In my own private curriculum-vitae, the injury done to me by diagnosed mental illness was assuming an increasingly disproportionate importance.

My year in the North Kensington house changed this relationship to mental illness. In essence it was a process of liberation. Within a few days of my arrival, it became clear that the strategies I had adopted during the previous two or three years would not be validated by the staff members at the house. The context within which I was dealing with life and its misfortunes was not going to be acknowledged wholesale and unchallenged. At my first meeting with my counsellor, the staff member who was to take particular interest in my progress, I opened up with a fairly exhaustive, and well-rehearsed, discourse on the limiting effects of manic depression in an uncaring society. The reaction was most unexpected: "That's all very interesting Peter. But it's in the past. I believe that you are able to change your life; to take responsibility for it, to take control of it. You don't have to be a victim. You have a lot of positive qualities, and we should find ways of using them." This may not appear exceptional. Indeed, in the light of the developments in social attitudes and techniques over the last ten years it may seem banal. But no one had spoken to me in those terms before. No psychiatrist had ever talked of the task in hand with anything approaching enthusiasm. It was the difference between listening to an explorer hacking back the encroaching jungle and hearing an orchard keeper talk of her estate. It was the difference between negative and positive impulsion.

In the simplest analysis, this was the most important lesson I absorbed during the time I spent at the Richmond Fellowship house: that the experience of "mental illness" need not be unreservedly negative, that changing to come to terms with such problems can be a positive, life-enhancing process, not a canker and a self-destruction, and above all that an individual may win control, remain in control, and not give himself up to "illness" and other opiate conceptions. It seems to me to be dangerously easy to lose one's perspective on "mental illness", particularly if one has spent periods of time in psychiatric care. I certainly had an erroneous perspective. Indeed, to some extent "mental illness" became my perspective, the high ground from which I surveyed my entire environment. I have met many people who have spent time inside psychiatric units of one kind or another. A large number would attest to the important psychological implications of being diagnosed and treated as "mentally ill". Almost all of these would, I believe, suggest that those implications are negative. It is certainly my impression that the chances that you will have problems involved in being "mentally-ill", as well as suffering from the symptoms of a "mental illness", are much increased by current psychiatric practice. It was in providing an antidote to such attitudes, and an alternative to my negative self-image, that my year in the therapeutic community was most significant.

Life in the community was all consuming. I was new to London. I had no alternative social focus. But even for those who came from the London area, the community became the most important focus for their lives. We tended to live an inward-facing life, looking in at our community life, looking into our own selves and our triumphs and disasters. In some respects, we were no less isolated than we would have been in a psychiatric unit. To a degree it was a hermetic existence. But at least it had a positive quality. It was very difficult not to become involved in the lives of those who shared your home. The quality of ships passing in the night which frequently pervades the admission ward was generally absent. We talked and listened a great deal – often late into the night. I think many of us believed we could support and change each other in these ways. Many of us were disheartened when things went wrong, and friends returned to hospital, or left the community altogether with their problems no closer to solution. It was inevitable that in such an intensive life-experience the ups and downs were heightened. Neutrality was a difficult option.

Things did not always go right. During my year at the house, numerous people overdosed, some massively. Someone attempted to cut his throat with a kitchen knife. Another jumped out of a first-floor window onto concrete and killed himself. In a tightly knit introspective community such events had an understandable impact, crystallising our hopes and fears and opening wide into the tissue of insecurity which clothed us all. The latter incident affected me in particular. I was the first person on the scene, ran for an ambulance to the hospital round the corner, and cleared up the blood afterwards. It was the first time I had seen a person dying. But more significantly it was the first time that someone I had known and not liked had committed suicide. I had never felt so implicated in the wrongness of the human condition as I did in the days following that death.

Not everyone was changed by their time in the community. I have subsequently met more than one fellow resident who looks back on his stay as a complete waste of time. A percentage of those who came into the house during my year there stayed for only a very short period, six or eight weeks perhaps, and then left. Amongst these there were a number who did not seem to be in a position to benefit from the therapeutic style being used in the community. Others, and those included many who remained for a year or even more, found change extremely difficult, if not impossible, and when they did eventually move on, did so with very mixed feelings. It is desperately difficult to change. When society, through its own definitions of the abnormal and the particularist partialities of its professional agencies, muddies the individual's field of operation, coherent action may be effectively precluded. The therapeutic community did at least offer some opportunity to those who wished to make the attempt at change.

Not everyone in therapeutic communities does wish to change, although such motivation was a supposed qualification for those who applied to the community in North Kensington. Individual residents that I knew clung to their defined positions with great tenacity. Sometimes this seemed to be due to a genuine desperation that any movement would mean disintegration, sometimes to outright defiance. In particular instances, such an attitude can provoke intense frustration and even anger among fellow community members. Frequently, I reacted as though my own position and prospects were being undermined. Nevertheless, in general it is hard to deny that psychiatry's rather clouded attitude to change as opposed to treatment or cure bears some responsibility. If the psychiatric approach gave rather more

49

emphasis to the positive potential of mental health rather than highlighting the disease and illness aspects of the phenomenon, individuals might have less excuse for avoiding an active approach to their predicaments. The identity of the so-called mentally ill, their integrity, their status as individual human beings and as valued members of contemporary society is under consistent erosion. It is perhaps hardly surprising that we should sometimes become defensive, reinforce our boundaries and declare "Here we stand. Death to the Invaders."

But for me the year from autumn 1973 to autumn 1974 was overwhelmingly positive. I was lucky insomuch as community life suited me and that I did not approach any manic crises while in the house. The belief that I was not merely a victim of a psychiatric history had been sown in me by my counsellor's attitude. It was reinforced by my ability to function as a valued member of the community. Within six weeks of my arrival, I had begun to train as a playgroup leader. By the time I left, I was working with preschool children and had secured my basic cer-tificate. Although the community was a very special, and to some extent artificial, society, it was a functioning unit and the first social environment I had encoun-tered in my adult life where I was able to play a positive and rewarding part. My competence had been under severe attack for several years, particularly from my own vantage point. Whatever I may, or may not, have been when I finally left the Richmond Fellowship house, I was at least increasingly aware of my own ability to avoid disintegration at the behest of incalculable influences I had once believed outside my control.

My arrival in London coincided with the blossoming of alternative therapies in the capital. Having experienced the broader approach offered by staff at the community, it seemed natural that I should try out some of the new techniques widely advertised in weekly magazines and newspapers. The atmosphere in the early 1970s was different from that of the middle 1980s. Alternative therapies had a novelty value in this country and I and others were undoubtedly influenced by the attractions of fashion. Over a decade later, I believe alternative therapies are viewed in a more sober manner, their true value and limitations more clearly per-ceived. I first joined therapy groups out of curiosity, because I was lonely and because, in a vague way, I believed that there might just be an alternative shortcut to happiness. I am certain that I am not the only one who has entered into such therapies with these uncertain motives. The belief that I might be plugging into an inner circuit to something was certainly very attractive.

The rules of the game in group therapies are somewhat different from the rules governing a therapeutic community. To some extent the game itself is dissimi-lar. Such at least is my experience. Over a period of three years starting in 1973, I was a member of encounter groups, gestalt therapy groups and on-going bio-energetics groups. In all these, regardless of how much I learnt and benefited, I was aware of a high degree of insecurity. I found one-off, or weekend, groups where the members were all strangers who would disappear in different directions at the end of the event particularly hard to handle. The context of a stable group of known and recognised individuals with which I was familiar from my experience in the community was quite absent here. The alternative therapies I experienced all encouraged the open expression of positive and negative emotions among the group. The power of the group as an agent for change was often revealed to great and beneficial effect. Nevertheless, with my own particular background, and in the absence of a stable and supportive group environment, the main lessons I learnt were in opposition to the general drift of the techniques employed.

In particular, I learnt to treat the idea that these special groups produced special insights with scepticism. I was continually being told that I was cold and intellectual by fellow group members, often within two hours of the session opening. It was some time before I convinced myself that this was not a true perception, but a judgement based largely on my physical appearance: tall and thin with John Lennon style glasses. In the same way, I began not to feel guilty about betraying the ideal when I refused to continue with a therapeutic exercise, despite the subtle goading of the group leader and the concerted pressure of the group. To establish my own position on the desirability of approved group behaviours like screaming, and bursting into tears, or frequent kissing and hugging, was also extremely difficult and, in retrospect, valuable. In a sense, I think I was always working myself away from group therapies, out of the alternative mould. However valuable the techniques may be – and bioenergetics, in particular, was useful for me – the veiled pressures alienated me. I have never taken easily to other people's advice, even more so if I am forced to respond to it spontaneously. My circumstances had led me into a great deal of being pushed around. In the final analysis, I felt that alternative therapies were repeating the same process in an infinitely more subtle way. It did not seem to be on my terms. Alternative therapies confirmed in me a new belief in my own resources. I emerged with a stronger resolve: to refuse to be pushed around some more.

At this time, it was impossible for me, and difficult for most who had similar experiences, to be unaware of contrasting scenarios that were offered regarding our predicament. Speaking baldly, one ascribed our mental health problems to illness, possibly even to the mechanisms of heredity. Certainly to factors which were largely outside our own control. The other implicated the social environment, our family circumstances, our inability to communicate satisfyingly with those around us. The dichotomy was, and is, quite marked. In-patients I knew were often quite opposed on what the real nature of our predicament was. Sometimes the day room would be split into clear and contrasted camps supporting one or other attitude. The more one studies the theories of causation and the research on which they are based, the more one finds the theorists and researchers hedging their bets. While the general public may believe that one day soon a giant pill will be found that can eradicate schizophrenia at one swallow, while many experts find it in their own interests to foster such beliefs, the actual evidence and the postulations which stem from it are closely guarded in sub clauses of qualification, paragraphs of academic caution. The exclusive validity of one approach against another is rarely asserted. When confronted in open academic debate the psychiatric professional is usually quite ready to vouchsafe contemporary ignorance.

But for the ordinary recipient of psychiatric provisions, it is all rather different. Whatever the subtleties of the academic argument may be, this individual will often have to face, as I did in the mid-1970s, two contrasting attitudes to his problems. Although there is no obvious reason why one should have to choose between one or the other, in reality there are quite often pressures to do just that. In the 1970s psychiatrists frequently dismissed alternative therapies, or psychotherapy, out of hand. I knew psychiatrists who made it as difficult as possible for their patients to explore alternatives to conventional psychiatry. Often the topic would be dismissed in one sentence at consultations. Sometimes it all had the feeling of heresy and the true believer. On the other hand, friends frequently attacked me when I admitted that I was using psychotropic drugs and reckoned I might continue to use them voluntarily for most of my life. The idea that I was willing not to be in control of myself and my life in a genuine way was often not accepted, except as an admission of a personal failure. The two approaches were becoming increasingly divergent. It was not easy for the individual to come to his own accommodation without at the same time assuming the total package offered by one or other extreme.

I believe it is important to recognise the implications of academic formulations for the ordinary person undergoing psychiatric care. In a sense we become the victims of these theories and philosophies at the same time as we become victims of so-called mental illness. An attitude to a problem is an integral part of the problem. Someone who feels that his illness is the result of a viral infection in childhood will often react differently to someone who believes his problem to be due to his upbringing and his inability to communicate with his peers. The area of mental distress is so complicated by social, political and moral overtones that it is particularly difficult for anyone to reach through to a healthy attitude. The polarisation of approaches which complicated my predicament in the mid-1970s still continues. The power residing in the concept of illness in its psychiatric context is such that many collapse into accepting it uncritically or react violently against the monotone construction that has been assembled around their lives.

1.06

DRUGS – THE MANY HEADED GUARD DOG

Barbiturates (type unknown); Valium (Diazepam); Librium (Chlordiazepoxide); Mogadon (Nitrazepam); Chloral Hydrate; Largactil (Chlorpromazine); Mellaril (Thioridazine); Depixol (Flupenthixol decanoate); Haldol (Haloperidol); Tryptizol (Amitriptyline); Lithium Carbonate; Kemadrin (drug to counteract side effects of some of the above drugs).

That is a list of the drugs that I have been prescribed at some time or other since I first came into contact with psychiatry. I cannot swear that it is comprehensive but, even so, I think it has a certain ring to it. Since the age of eighteen, I have been consuming one or more of these drugs – sometimes as many as four at once – with little interruption. Whether this reveals me as being dependent on drugs, I'm not completely certain. What it does indicate is the massive reliance – one might almost say dependence – of psychiatry on drugs to tackle the problems of those who stray within its portals.

No consideration of the role played by chemotherapy in contemporary psychiatry can proceed without recognising at the outset the revolution chemotherapy has affected on psychiatric practice since the 1950s. At the same time, no one should be unaware of the historical evidence that revolutions frequently leave in their wake new tyrannies as great and stubborn as those they have swept away. The possibility that psychiatry may have found the bathwater but drowned the baby is not an idle fancy.

Chemotherapy has been the great controller within psychiatry. Without chemotherapy, I do not believe we should have the open door policy which now motivates care in many psychiatric hospitals. Although the principles of the open-door approach may have pre-dated the widespread use of mood altering drugs, it is inconceivable to me that most in-patients today would be living on open wards had not such drugs provided the carers with the means to manage, and control, without the harsher forms of compulsion and incarceration. On a personal level, I acknowledge the fact that had I been born 20 years earlier, I would have spent long periods in padded cells and straitjackets. Indeed, I might not have easily survived my grosser periods of mania had I become adult before the chemotherapy revolution. In the broadest sense, chemotherapy has restricted the starker dimensions of mental distress.

DOI: 10.4324/9781003636434-9

If the boundaries of personal suffering, the quality of life within the psychiatric hospital, have been modified by the introduction of drug treatments, so too has the general condition of life for the so-called mentally ill within society as a whole. Nowadays, even those who are judged to be suffering from the most severe and recalcitrant psychotic illnesses will not necessarily spend the best part of their lives inside institutions. People do not disappear into bins for years and decades with quite the same frequency as was common 30 or 40 years ago. Undoubtedly, this is in large part due to the controlling power of chemotherapy. While we may credit ourselves as having built a more liberal and more permissive society since the 1930s, I think it is foolish to believe that had chemotherapy not been able to temper the grosser misbehaviours of the so-called mentally ill, they would not be precisely where they were in those days. And liberal society would be looking in and going tut-tut.

So, chemotherapy has made the possibility of an accommodation between this disadvantaged, this feared minority and the wider society more real. The patent uncontrollability which makes this group such an unattractive package to the general public has now been massaged closer to the mainstream boundaries of acceptability. Without chemotherapy, there would not even be the illusion that we are waving to each other from the same platform. On a personal level, quite apart from the elimination of much distress, the use of mood-changing drugs has enabled many people to live their life, or most of it, within the boundaries of the wider society. To some degree our lives have become more acceptable to ourselves as well as becoming more acceptable to others. Exactly where such a balance lies, and the degree to which chemotherapy weighs it to one side or another, are vitally important political, social and personal questions. I shall discuss them below. In the meantime, I would like to record that whatever reconciliation I have made between myself and my problems, between myself with my problems and the non-accepting society in which I try to live, has been achieved with the assistance of chemotherapy. Although I have close friends who will say the exact opposite, I believe that drug treatment has been helpful to me, and I feel that my progress through the last eighteen years would have been at certain times considerably more traumatic had it not been for the ministrations of mood-changing drugs. Furthermore, regardless of our individual experiences, I would maintain that any recipient of psychiatric provisions who is not aware that chemotherapy has been responsible in large part for winning us such power as we presently have over our position in society is fooling himself and ignoring the historical drive which activates our cause.

It is not possible to permit people to live within the wider community of their contemporaries, to treat them like dirt and then expect no comeback. If you keep people locked away in isolated institutions for fifteen or 20 years, they will likely end up accepting whatever happens to be dumped on them. They may have no clear idea of, or consistent contact with, a better deal. They have probably forgotten what the inside of a Woolworth's looks like, let alone what respect and self-direction implies. They cannot have the means to pursue their expectations. Perhaps they do not even have the expectations. But to give those who formerly would have been long-term inmates, the advantage of living their lives in the same settings as their peers, and then to disadvantage them, is something else again. You cannot tell someone that he can join the party, and then expect him to sit on the rug with his legs crossed all night. If you believe that you are alright, and you are sharing the same space as those who say they are alright, how can you accept it when they treat you otherwise? Once the door is open, it's too late for the hosts to change the menu. It's no longer possible, in my opinion, to believe that the so-called mentally ill will not win in the end. And we have chemotherapy to thank for opening the door.

Part 2

HOLDING IT ALL TOGETHER, 1983–2000

2.00

INTRODUCTION TO PART 2

Nutters get
Compulsory sunsets.
Wall to wall landscaping of the soul.
Always a rugged coast, salt-flecked but liveable.
Always a hero looking west,
Going on about the forward march of science.
[From 'Drugtime Cowboy Joe' (1991) in: *Brown*
Linoleum Green Lawns, Hearing Eye, 2006]

The keynote of this selection is the astonishing diversity of writing here, in subject matter and genre, including: '*We're Not Mad, We're Angry*', an acclaimed dramatic script for television from 1986, with an accompanying commentary [2.02 and 2.03], with echoes of '*In Two Minds*' (1967) and '*Family Life*' (1971), produced by Tony Garnett and directed by Ken Loach; a series of published letters in *OpenMind* magazine between 1983 and 1985 that exemplify Peter's growing critical awareness and the heightened politicisation of his stance [2.01]; various imaginative pieces, including the Melvin Menz cartoons by 'Niall' [2.04]; and a number of reflective pieces of the first order on the affinity of spiritual crises with madness [2.12], and on the significance of psychosis, notably '*Valuing Psychosis: A Personal View*' [2.14], a landmark essay from 1994, previously unpublished, that has only recently been discovered among Peter's writings that offers a compelling statement and overview, based on Peter's experience in the mental health system over the previous 27 years, of the demeaning treatment meted out to users who have the temerity to attribute some measure of value to their experience of psychosis. In 'Through the Revolving Door' [2.15] Peter reflects on how the psychiatric acute ward that for the past fifteen years has seemed to him a place where nothing was really happening might be given a new lease of life.

Looking back on her experience at the legendary *Survivors Speak Out* Edale Conference in 1987, which played a formative role in the development of the mental health survivor movement, with Lorraine Bell as co-ordinator and Peter Campbell as

DOI: 10.4324/9781003636434-11

secretary, mental health user consultant Mary Nettle recalled in 2006 how the conference was 'a most amazing experience. A great array of ideas was expressed, and there was Peter Campbell holding it all together. We need people who can do that.... That's what we need within the user movement; we've got to be able to embrace diversity in all senses'. 'Holding it all together' and embracing diversity: in these astute remarks Mary Nettle (2006) aptly highlights the creative energy and direction that Peter succeeded in bringing across these critical years from 1983 to 2000.

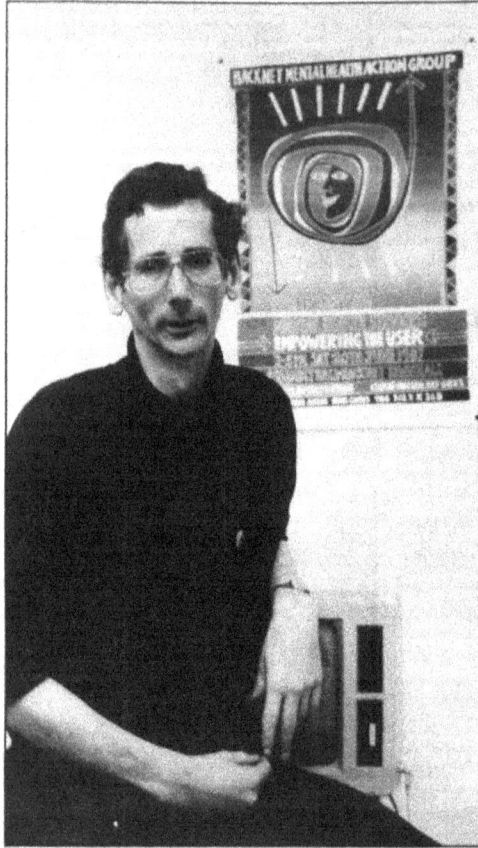

● Ex-patient Peter Campbell: "The programme was deliberately provocative."

©Newsquest Media Group

To exemplify this diverse creative energy, we include three mental health cartoons from the Melvin Menz series that Peter created for the newsletters of *Survivors Speak Out* [2.04].

The section concludes with several brief extracts [2.17–2.22; see also 3.01 and 3.04] taken from an extensive video life story recording with Peter in 2000, interviewed by Pete Fleischmann, one of 50 comprising the *Mental Health Testimony Archive*. The archive is now publicly accessible at the British Library [see Resources page below]. Peter was central to this groundbreaking oral history project, initiated by Mental Health Media and run by, and for, those who had experienced mental health service provision in the UK. Rob Perks, then Oral History Curator at the British Library, was an advisor to the project. Peter's Testimony 2000 interview engages with a range of topics such as his discovery on returning to Cambridge after his first breakdown that becoming a mental patient involves falling out of a familiar world; his experience of seclusion and of being put on section; and his reflections on a period at a therapeutic community, the Richmond Fellowship (RF). Though for many years he had thought of himself as a mental patient, and latterly as a community mental patient, at the RF Peter becomes aware that an alternative destiny may, after all, still be open to him. Though eventually it was eclipsed by his commitment to the emerging psychiatric survivor movement, he shares the huge importance that his work with pre-school children held for him over many years, briefly succeeding in the formative years between 1983 and 1989 in combining his work with children and with adult user groups [see also 2.08]. Peter's Testimony 2000 interview is © British Library and these extracts are used with permission.

In Peter's profound misgivings at 2.18 [see also 3.12 and 3.13] over seclusion as a euphemism for solitary confinement are vivid echoes of a history of dissension, still alive today as Peter evokes, reaching back to the 1830s and before. Asylum reformer John Conolly (1794–1866) strongly favoured seclusion (his preferred term) as a practical remedy in asylums if it was properly monitored and temporary, objecting that it was falsely labelled as solitary confinement, though his opponents alleged that it was exactly that, blurring the distinction between treatment and punishment (Ignatieff, 1989; Topp, 2018).

In the 1980s, Peter was also experimenting with writing for young children, crafting a series of stories with titles such as *The Monster Who Could Only Smile*, with a comical wise man and themes of social control and expectations, *The Bloob, the Smurg and the Koog*, which deals with emotions, *Big Red* and *Beth the Vandal*. To give readers a taste of these creations, we have found space for *Big Red,* which we have placed at the end of the book just before the Afterwords. Alongside the children's writings are stories for an older readership, three of which we reproduce here in abridged form, *Madness Café, Nutter's Diary* and *Hotel Galactica*. In many respects, Peter's adult imaginative writing bridges the gap between adult and infantile experience. 'Do the children know they are keeping me alive, I wonder?' asks the narrator in *Nutter's Diary.* Infantile experience, blocked toilets and poetic inspiration spill into each other. The toilet was not working, but the 'poem just flowed out and I felt good' [2.06].

In his early writing, Peter quite frequently enlisted Niall, his middle name, as a pseudonym, though later he appears to have distanced from Niall. When one of us introduced his middle initial into the byline of an article, Peter asked him to strike it out. In several of these pieces, cafés occupy a central place, as they did in Peter's own life, both for the pleasures of eating and for their sociality. Peter had a favourite café in Cricklewood where for many years he used to meet with other survivor friends, and at Napsbury Psychiatric Hospital, where Peter was quite frequently a resident, there were the pleasures of the *Double D*, just outside the hospital gates, where you could get 'a proper greasy spoon meal' [3.07]. At Hotel Galactica ('there's no Hotel Recommended sign on the doorpost'), Micah, a fellow resident, remarks to Niall, the narrator: 'You were a long way out last night'. 'I suppose so and they were giving me a good wee push too' rejoins Niall. 'Micah nodded. "Doing the Magellan" he said, and we both laughed'. Drug-assisted or not, 'doing the Magellan' is seemingly a figure for travels outside consensual reality that held some lasting significance for Peter for he deployed it subsequently as the title for a detailed series of notes and drafts that he compiled between 1997 and 2004 (not reproduced here but available in the PCLP archive) in which, among other concerns, he reflects critically on the supposed incommensurability of psychotic experience. 'Emphasis on isolating and separating nature of psychotic thought, feeling etc. How much of this is due to essential incomprehensibility etc of experience and how much to not having easy access to frameworks of understanding? Is psychiatry trying to make the content of a psychotic episode communicable or actually going the opposite way of separating it off?'

References

Ignatieff, Michael (1989) *A Just Measure of Pain: The Penitentiary in the Industrial Revolution 1750–1850*, London: Penguin

Nettle, Mary (2006). 'Mary's Story', in: Marion Clark & Tony Glynn eds., '*Two Decades of Change: Celebrating User Involvement*', pdf accessible at: http://studymore.org.uk/twodec.pdf

Topp, Leslie (2018) 'Single Rooms, Seclusion and the Non-Restraint Movement in British Asylums, 1838–1844', *Social History of Medicine*, 31 (4): 679–700.

2.01

PUBLISHED LETTERS TO
OpenMind MAGAZINE

OpenMind 3. jabs & pills [c 1983]

Madam, I am a manic depressive and have had nearly fifteen years of admission and re-admission into N.H.S. psychiatric hospitals. Now, at the age of 34, I am in control of my illness so that long admissions are not necessary. Recently I was in an area where I had been a regular in-patient over a period of ten years. I had left my Priadel at home and was prevailed upon by a relative to seek some temporary medication to get me through the night.

I went to the hospital where I am well-known. I asked for two Mogadon. These were refused, so I asked for Valium but was offered Largactil. I said Largactil gave me a lot of side effects so they said I could be admitted overnight on Valium. In the next two hours, I received two intra-muscular injections of some substance, the latter of which I strenuously resisted. Next morning, I discharged myself. I was not told what drug I had been injected with. Indeed, when returning the following week to make a complaint, it became clear that the staff themselves might not be able to establish what drug I had been forced to digest, and from whose side effects I had been given no protection. Is this a normal response to a request for a couple of hypnotic tablets?

OpenMind 4. coming through [c.1983]

Madam, I was delighted to read 'Coming Through' in *OpenMind 2*. I am a manic depressive of fifteen years standing and went through the same mental hospital, Richmond Fellowship and therapy process as Naomi.

Now I no longer feel the need for such support but am well aware, as a victim of a recurrent illness, of the need to be always well-armed against relapses. It is vital for all mentally ill and manic-depressive people in particular, to be aware of some of the practical and physical problems in negotiating a relapse 'successfully'. I feel it is foolish for us to ignore the possibilities of future problems and also not to realize that the right sort of help is often not available in times of crisis.

In order to 'stay through' despite setbacks, I believe we must become conscious of how we can manage our own breakdowns and put concerted pressure on the

DOI: 10.4324/9781003636434-12

N.H.S. to provide us with sensitive support. It is our own fault if we succumb to state psychiatry's facile resort to the God of Chemotherapy in every admission. If mental patients never use their voices, is it any wonder that doctors only use our throats for pill-swallowing?

OpenMind 6. professional imperialism

Madam, recently on television, Tessa Jowell, an assistant director of MIND, spoke of the need to share the decision-making process with the mentally ill themselves. These sentiments have been expressed in public before and have sometimes surfaced in the magazines and publications of MIND. It is hoped that on this occasion the ideal will be enthusiastically pursued.

For example, the balance of *OpenMind* itself seems to be heavily weighted in favour of the expert. Much of the advertising would seem to support this view. Thus, *OpenMind* reflects rather than confronts the division between the professional and the consumer. It is my view that it is inadequate to confine the voice of the ordinary person to a letters column.

The arrogant assumption that the mentally ill never analyse the significance of their experience or are incapable of conveying it to other sections of society should be directly challenged by MIND. Sooner or later, someone is going to take the plunge.

OpenMind 8. regaining control

Madam, in his article in *OpenMind 6*, Richard Jameson raised the question of why so many people are reluctant to take drugs and why they believe coming off medication is an achievement. This is indeed an important question underlined by the high percentage of psychotropic drug users who do give up their medication soon after returning to the community.

As Richard Jameson points out, drugs may validly be seen as chemicals the body needs. Such a viewpoint is rational but takes no account of the context within which psychotropic drugs are prescribed. It is the presentation of drug treatment which is the problem. Drugs are designed to help but they often are the target of resentment because they are not prescribed in an atmosphere of open helpfulness and because they become the only form of help consistently offered. This is one way in which they may appear to be an obstacle to the patients' real needs and therefore take on the guise of punishment.

Loss of control is a central element in the experience of the mentally ill. The ways in which drug treatments are presented often prove inimical to our needs for regaining control. The secrecy surrounding the side effects and other implications of drug treatment does not help in this respect. I accept my own need to take lithium for the foreseeable future. The achievement is not to come off drugs but to win back self-control of one's life. To this end, the current overreliance of the N.H.S. on drug treatments and drug-oriented philosophies can sometimes prove an obstacle.

OpenMind 15. the work ethic

Madam, for many years the idea that chemotherapy assisted by occupational and industrial therapies would prepare the individual for return to productive life in the community, was an established truth – as many N.H.S. consumers found to their cost in the 60s and 70s. In recent times it has become clear to a much broader range of people that to offer employment as a goal of rehabilitation is cynical to say the least. The expectations which were peddled to mental patients in the 60s and 70s can now be seen as threadbare. It is time the psychiatric establishment reassessed the goals of the processes they supervise.

Perhaps it would be appropriate to examine the whole ethic upon which rehabilitation lies. Certainly, it is my experience that neither occupational nor industrial therapies satisfactorily meet the needs of those returning to the community. Until the experts accept that the needs of the consumer do not fit, indeed may never have fitted, into the preconceptions of their service, it is the mental patient who will continue to pay the penalties.

OpenMind 17. ECT: feared

It was interesting to read Mr McDowell's defence of ECT and to note the very specific area within which he defended its use. My own experience makes me sceptical as to whether ECT is only being used on those who fall within such defined limits.

There are two other aspects of ECT which are of some importance. Firstly, the role that ECT plays in the psychology and mythology of in-patient life. It would be interesting to know what patients and staff of admission wards, for example, feel like, knowing that such a treatment is on the menu. I know that on my first admission in the 1960s it took me less than ten days to develop an insistent fear of ECT even though there was no prospect of my being treated with it at that time.

Second, it is crucial to consider the presentation of ECT to the prospective user. As with other treatments, it seems the user is frequently not given the full picture – -either on the possible side effects, the limits of benefit or the alternatives which exist. I do not believe that the use of ECT is always approached with honesty, nor that sensitive support is always offered to patients who face this treatment. ECT is greatly feared. By refusing to face this openly, professionals treat users in a manner whose effects are as damaging as the more easily quantifiable effects of the treatment itself.

OpenMind 18. advocacy

In the light of Bob Sang's article (*OpenMind* 17), it is perhaps worthwhile to consider MIND's role as advocate on behalf of the mentally ill.

There are many people who do not wish MIND to speak on their behalf. They are capable and willing to speak for themselves without the intervention of a professional body as interpreter. Indeed, some of their continuing dissatisfaction is because many agencies, including MIND, are so lukewarm in allowing them direct access or voice. To such a group, the trumpeted position of advocate is more of an obstacle than an avenue. It seems MIND wants to run things on their terms. It is MIND for the mentally ill, not MIND with the mentally ill.

My second major concern is that advocacy will only act as a cement for the system in which it operates. Whatever the commitment of the players, the game is still the same and the reserve team is highly unlikely to be allowed on the pitch. MIND bestrides the field of mental health and says it is our advocate. I think it is time MIND sharpened up its ideas of what it can and cannot, will and will not, do. Then perhaps the rest of us would have a better chance of a go.

2.02

WE'RE NOT MAD, WE'RE ANGRY (1986)

GP surgery

The voice

Alice Bell is a mother of two in her early 30s. She is married. Her husband has recently got a job away from their hometown, forcing Alice to move away from family and friends. Recently he has begun to work on the night shift.

Her voice will be largely classless. Her diagnosis will be depression.

Alice monologue:	I wasn't sure about going to see the doctor but I couldn't think what else to do I just needed somebody to help me sort things out.

Doctor is busy writing at desk.

Scarcely looking up, doctor says:	Sit down please.

Doctor continues to write busily.

Doctor, picking up sheaf of notes:	Mrs Graham…?
Alice:	Bell, doctor, Alice Bell
Doctor:	Oh Yes. I've been given the wrong notes Hang on now.

Doctor gets up and goes over to the filing cabinet turning his back on Alice. Begins to search through files.

> Umm now, er Bell, um Begazelle, Begley, now
> Bell, Alice.

He removes the file and begins to read.

Plucking up courage to plunge into an explanation, Alice speaks.

Alice:	I've been feeling really bad recently. I can't seem to keep up with things at home like I used to before… it's like… I can't…

DOI: 10.4324/9781003636434-13

Doctor:	(not hearing Alice properly and returning to the desk with cor-rect notes)
	sorry hang on a minute
	looking at notes
	now we haven't seen you for some time now, have we? How are the…
	(looking at file)
	headaches, did the er….
	(looks at file)
	Migralibe sort the problem out for you?
Alice:	It's not the migraine it's just I seem to feel so tired these days and things mount up.
	I'm stuck indoors every day my husband's on the nights now, we never see him, he tells me to pull myself together but I just can't seem to, I need someone to talk to, but I never get out to meet anyone now, not since we moved.
Doctor:	I see. How are you sleeping?
Alice:	Not too well. If I could just get away. I feel so shut in. Some-times I think if I could just get away for a day or two things would be clearer.
Doctor:	What about meals? Are you eating properly?
Alice:	No not really
Doctor:	I see.
Alice:	I eat the same as the children. It's easiest.
Doctor:	Perhaps but not necessarily the best. Now I think you need something to calm you down a little, relax you, help you sleep a bit better (starts to write prescription).
Alice:	It's the children. If I could just get out on my own for a change.
Doctor:	Couldn't your mother help you out?
Alice:	It's not that easy, not since we moved.
Doctor:	OK look, I'm going to try you on these, they should help. You'll be able to sort things out now… get back to normal. But if you have any problems come right back and we'll see what we can do….OK?
Alice:	Thank you……. Goodbye.
	(Doctor writes up notes)
Alice monologue:	I took the Valium. They didn't seem to help. I just felt more tired. A couple of months later I locked myself in the bedroom. I felt I had to be alone. The doctor came. He told my husband it will be best for me to go into hospital.

Scene. Admission Interview
A nursing station in an admission ward.
Hospital 1: admission

68

Charge nurse at desk in background busy at filing cabinet.
   Alice enters and sits down at desk opposite charge nurse.

Alice monologue:	He said I'd only be in for a few days. That just being here would help. But I couldn't see how.
Charge:	Your husband has given us some details already. We just need one or two more. I forgot to ask him if you had a phone at home. Have you got a telephone?
Alice:	Seven three seven. Seven seven three eight.
Charge:	Is that double seven three eight?
Alice:	Yes.
Charge:	Right. Now.
	(Looks down his form)
Alice:	Will I see a doctor soon?
Charge:	[to student nurse]. No. Jackie. The yellow form. In the third drawer. Behind the 136 forms. That's it.
	(Takes form to Alice.)
	Now what about next of kin?
	Your husband?
Charge:	Alice? It's your husband isn't it?
Alice:	Is it blood? Blood kin? There's my mother.
Charge:	I'll put your husband down. It's just a formality.
Charge:	Now it's just religion. C of E?
Charge:	Shall I put down C of E then?
Alice:	No. I haven't been baptized.
Charge.	Alright. I'll leave it.
Alice:	I'm worried about Carol and Barry. I don't think my husband can cope.
	He's not very good with the children you know.
	Phone on desk rings interrupting them. Charge nurse picks it up and listens.
Charge on phone:	No, no, I can't Peter……..look, just tell her she's got to take it….no, no tell her….Oh I know, yea, yea. Really, God that bloody woman thinks this place is a hotel…..what, no, no. Look Nigel knows his appointments have been cancelled, he's just playing games….OK. Right…yes 24…..no hang on, 25 with this new admission. Right.
	(Puts phone down. Turning to Alice.)
	Now, where were we? Oh yes! The social worker will be dropping in, Alice, I'm sure. Don't worry yourself. Think about getting better, that's the main Thing. Now did you bring your clothes with you?
Student nurse:	She has an overnight case here.
Charge:	Good. That's fine.

Charge:	We like all the new patients to take a bath and change into their night clothes. It's more comfortable for them. Just for today.
Alice:	But it's lunchtime.
Charge:	I know. Jackie will take you along when you've done.
	(Alice picks up bag.)
	No leave your bag here.
	We'll have to do a property check later.....It's for safety's sake you know.
Student Nurse:	Come on Alice. I'll come down to the bathroom with you, OK?
Alice:	But I don't need a bath.
	(Alice and Student Nurse go out.)
Alice:	They gave me a bath. The nurse just stood over me......It was as if they expected me to do something. I felt so embarrassed.

The ward

Alice comes into the day room of the ward for the first time, dressed in nightclothes and dressing gown just as lunchtime medication has begun.

Hospital 2: The ward

Noises of ward on soundtrack. Camera moves into room towards nurse and charge nurse by unopened drugs trolley. Four patients sit nearby. There is one vacant chair.
    One patient, David, is wandering.

Alice [monologue]:	After I had had a bath I sat on my bed for a while. I felt so stupid....dressed in my nightclothes at lunchtime.
Student nurse to Alice:	There that looks much better.
	We'll give you some tablets in a moment.
	That dressing gown goes quite well, doesn't it?
	You look much fresher now.
	(Student nurse retires towards drugs trolley. Charge nurse steps forward and ushers Alice to the vacant chair in the group.)
Charge nurse:	Come and sit here Alice.
	(Introducing Alice to others in the group.)
	This is Ajay, Eileen, Norma and Sarah.
	Sarah will look after you. Won't you Sarah?
Patient [Pat] Sarah:	What?
	(Looks up, then nods towards Alice.
	Charge nurse returns to trolley. While this is happening Patient Norma, who is a bit 'sleepy', looks over at Alice.)

Pat Norma:	Hullo. Just come in? Did you have your lunch?
	(Alice nods.)
	Meanwhile, charge nurse has opened trolley. Charge nurse and student nurse begin to dispense medication.
Charge (in cheerful voice):	Medication everyone!
Pat David, who is now standing near chairs:	Largactil, Haloperidol, Kemadrin, that's me. What are you?
Charge:	Come on, David. You first.
	David goes over to trolley without delay. Medication is dispensed.
Student nurse:	Largactil 250, Haloperidol? Kemadrin? There we are.
	(Charge nurse signs along the cardex.)
Student nurse:	Sarah, come for your tablet please.
Pat Sarah:	They make me tired. That's why I can't do OT.
Student nurse:	Come on love. Take them now. You've been so much better.
Pat Sarah:	No!
Charge:	Oh, come on Sarah, you know if you don't take them like this we'll have to give you them by injection. You don't want that again.
	(Sarah takes them.)
	It's good for you to get off the ward Sarah, you know that. Look at Ajay. Ajay gets a lot of benefit from OT don't you Ajay?
Pat Ajay:	Yes Mon Kapitain!
	Patient Ajay gets up and goes towards drugs trolley. Student dispenses his drugs.
Pat Sarah:	[looks at Alice]. We know………We know
	(Camera starts to pan away around ward. Noises in background.)
Alice monologue:	My husband came to see me in the evening. He said 'I don't want no wife of mine in this mad house!' I didn't reply.

Consultant interview

Alice monologue:	I didn't feel any better for sitting around on the ward. They said the consultant would sort things out for me. I waited two days to see him.
	(Alice enters consulting room. Consultant is seated at desk.)

71

Consultant:	Sit down please Mrs Bell.
	(Alice sits down.)
Consultant:	I'm doctor Bakewell. I'll be dealing with your case. I may not be able to see you every time. In which case Dr Patel, my registrar, will be seeing you. I believe you were seen by the duty doctor when you first came in, Dr Capstick.
	(Alice no reply.)
Consultant:	You have met Dr Capstick Mrs. Bell? He saw you when you first came in.
Alice:	The young doctor. He spoke to me. He didn't say very much.
Consultant:	That's right. Well, how do you feel now? Since coming in?
Alice:	I don't know really. I'm worried about being away from home.
Consultant:	You seem to be a bit tense. Let's see. Have you slept better since you came in?
Alice:	Not really doctor. They brought someone in yesterday. She was crying all night. I wasn't able to sleep much at home but in here it's worse.
Consultant:	Yes it is sometimes difficult to sleep in a dormitory at first. Now Dr Capstick says that you feel things have been building up to this for the last three or four months. Do you feel this?
Alice:	Yes for at least three or four months. It's been some time.
Consultant:	So it's the family really. Nothing else?
Alice:	Well, the family is not everything.
Consultant:	No, no ….Now Alice, do you remember locking yourself in the bedroom?
Alice:	Yes
Consultant:	Hmm…. Dr Capstick says you locked yourself in the bedroom and wouldn't come out.
Alice:	Yes I couldn't stand it anymore. I just wanted to be alone for a bit.
Consultant:	You er….er….. didn't want to harm yourself?
Alice:	No, I just wanted to get away from things.
Consultant:	Yes I see. Has there been a history of mental illness in your family Mrs Bell, as far as you know?
Alice:	No, not as far as I know….. Ohh my husband has always said one of my uncles was a bit strange.
Consultant:	I see, in what way?
Alice:	Ohh I don't know, he was just a bit shy I guess, but he seemed OK to me.
Consultant:	Fine. Have you ever felt so…..down in the dumps before?
Alice:	Not as bad as this.
Consultant:	I see. But you have felt something like this?
Alice:	No not really. I think it's just the way we live and where we live.

Consultant:	Yes. Well, you certainly seem a bit wound up at the moment. I think I'll just adjust your medication a little.
Consultant:	Take the edge off your anxiety. Then I'll get Dr Patel to come and have a chat with you tomorrow. Get a few more details... sort things out for you.
	Right... now, just don't worry.
Alice:	Thanks.
Alice monologue:	I wanted to tell him that I knew why I felt so depressed but there just didn't seem to be the time. In the last six weeks I only saw him twice.

Industrial therapy

Alice monologue:	For the past four weeks they tried to teach me how to cook in what they called occupational therapy. I told them they were wasting my time and theirs. The last thing I needed were domestic science lessons. They said they'd try me on something new.

Hospital 4: Therapy

Alice enters the industrial therapy room and approaches instructor who is sitting at his desk.

Instructor looks up.

Alice:	I'm Alice Bell. Birch Ward. I've come for industrial therapy.
Instructor:	Fine then Alice. I'll be with you in a minute.

Alice looks around. One of the patients on the cotton wool ball packing line notices her.

Patient Norma (ironically):	We're cotton picking! Alice.....
	(Alice does not reply. Continues to look.)
Instructor (from out of shot):	OK love. Come and sit on that chair, won't you?

Alice Bell goes and sits at vacant chair. Instructor goes and stands opposite across the table and is standing by patient Eileen. In the following sequence, patient Eileen is 'taking the Mickey', ever so gently of course, out of the instructor.

Instructor:	I'll explain what we're doing here. It's cotton balls as you see. Picking and packing. OK? It's not difficult but some people do find it tricky, so we'll take it slowly.
	Eileen's been here some time now. She knows. Eh Eileen?

73

Patient Eileen (leaning towards
Alice and making a face):   It's not very difficult Alice.

As instructor explains the work, patient Eileen does it with maximum efficiency – in a mocking way.

Instructor: You take the cotton wool here you see. You separate it into small bundles and put it into the bags, so now you must ensure each bag is fairly tightly packed. You'll find that 27 balls fill the bag. Then place the bags on your left with the open end facing towards you. There we are. No…no…. I'm sorry to my left hand, your right hand… then someone else takes the little bags and pops them into large boxes. They tie them up first of course. And that's the system, my love.

Instructor's actions have brought the assembly line to halt.
    Patient Ajay and patient David appear at instructor's side.

Patient Ajay (with
  exaggerated urgency):   Mister Downs. Mister Downs.
Patient David: No more little bags left.
Instructor: I'll be with you in a minute.
To Alice: OK then Alice?
Patient Eileen: We don't strain ourselves for £7.83 a week.
Instructor: You can have an overall if you wish. We like to keep the place tidy looking. We'll be having a tea break in twenty minutes.
    (Patient David gets up and walks out.)
Instructor: David, where are you off to? I've told you, no smoking in the toilet.
    Alice looks around.
Alice monologue: Every day I worked there for five hours. It was therapeutic but not in the way they intended. They said the drugs weren't helping. They said I needed ECT to Lift my depression. I didn't want to sign the consent form but they talked me into it. They said it was for the best.
    (Atmosphere noises of waiting room)
Student nurse: Alice please!
    Alice approaches bed.
    (Student nurse towards Alice, helping)
Student nurse: OK Alice now. Just slip onto the bed. It's all right.
    There's nothing to be frightened of.

	(Alice slips onto the bed.)
Student nurse:	That's fine. Now just lie down. Relax. The doctor won't be a minute.
	(Sound of the anaesthetist approaching and the treatment trolley.)
Student nurse:	This is Alice Bell.
Anaesthetist:	Hello Alice. You're all right then?
Student nurse:	She's been very good.
Anaesthetist:	Have you had an anaesthetic before Alice?
Alice:	Yes.
Anaesthetist:	Good. Well, it's just the same. You won't feel anything at all. You'll have a little sleep. When you wake up, it will all be over. Very easy these days.
Alice:	Yes, they said.
Anaesthetist:	I'm just going to do a couple of checks. I'll just have a listen to your heart. Fine, good, good.
Anaesthetist:	OK Alice. Now are you wearing any hair pins, chains, that sort of thing?
Alice:	No.
Anaesthetist:	That's lovely. OK.
To student nurse:	She seems a bit anxious.
Looking at drug sheet:	Did they give her any PRN Valium on the ward?
Student nurse:	Yes
Anaesthetist:	Fine….. OK Alice now we're just going to pop this in your mouth
	Biting bar inserted.
	Now, you'll just feel a little prick on the back of your hand.
Alice:	I'm not too sure about this.
Anaesthetist:	Look Alice, Dr Bakewell knows which treatment is most appropriate for your condition. There's nothing to worry about. It's perfectly safe. We do hundreds every week…. You won't feel a thing.
	(Alice loses consciousness. Fade out. This is followed by a fade up as Alice wakes in recovery room.)
Student nurse:	OK Alice? It's all over. Are you OK Alice?
	(Alice doesn't reply.)
	Yes, you're alright. I expect you're feeling a bit woozy. Put your slippers on and we'll go back to the ward. They would have kept some breakfast for you.
Alice:	I've had breakfast. I've got a terrible headache.
	Was I here before?

Student nurse:	Yes, you were. Don't worry about the head.
	It's probably just the anaesthetic. It does make you feel a bit odd. You'll be OK when it wears off.
Alice:	I feel so strange. Where are my slippers?
Student nurse:	Right here. Right at the foot of your bed.
	Come on let's go back to the ward.
Alice (ironically):	The ECT helped my depression. For a few days I
	Couldn't remember why I was depressed.

Discharge
Scene: The Consultant's Office

Alice monologue:	I didn't think being in the hospital was doing me any good. I was getting too used to their routine.
	I felt I was ready to go home…. Eventually so did They.
Consultant:	Well, I think it's time we should be thinking of sending you home don't you? Now, we know you may not feel quite ready yet. But you've really come on a great deal while you've been here.
	Nowadays we don't believe in keeping people in hospital any longer than is absolutely necessary.
	Often it just doesn't help. We don't want people to get bogged down in here. It's not necessary. It's not like the old days. With the kind of treatments we have now, we're able to look after people in the community, in their own homes. It's better all round. It seems you have settled down a bit. The Medication is working quite nicely now. I think it's helped you to get things under control….and the shock treatment has pulled you up a bit…good….And I understand from the social worker that she sorted things out for you at home. So….. we should be thinking in terms of getting you back to your husband, getting you er….back to normal. You want to be back home with the children, don't you Mrs Bell?
Alice:	I guess so.
Consultant:	That's right, but don't worry we won't be leaving you on your own…. If you've got any problems nip along to your GP, Doctor, er er….
	[Refers to notes]
	Kael.
	I'll be dropping him a line…. And of course Mrs…..er Blyth, the social worker will be looking in on you from time to time…to see er…..that you are alright. You'll find there is a whole system of support outside these days. Just because we

	have to bring you in this time doesn't mean we should ever have to again…. quite the contrary……. You know, sometimes I think we psychiatrists will be doing ourselves out of a job. I hope we won't see each other again, Mrs Bell.
	Goodbye.
Alice:	Thanks.
Alice monologue:	That afternoon my husband came to take me home.
	He said he was glad to have me back. He said it was difficult to cope with everything without me there. He said that now we could get back to normal.

[It may be of value to have the link to the YouTube extract of the film of *We're Not Mad, We're Angry*, which includes a brief comment from a youthful Peter Campbell: https://www.youtube.com/watch?v=qD36m1mveoY]

2.03

BLEAK READING ON JUDGEMENT DAY

by Peter Campbell	*ON AIR OFF AIR*, November 1986
	FOCUS

The history of man's response to madness will make bleak reading on judgement day. For centuries, the mad were driven out of cities, chained by neck and foot in dungeons or burnt at the stake as witches. Since the onset of civilization, we have either lived beyond the pale altogether or been locked up in romantic garrets. But now it is the 20th century and madness is no more. Instead, there is mental illness. And to combat it there is psychiatry – a new dynamic expertise, a branch of established medical science. Now, it would seem, the old story has been irreversibly changed.

In fact, the position of the so-called mentally ill remains unenviable. Although no longer openly persecuted, we are marginalized, discriminated against when we seek employment, forced to live within an entirely negative context. Everywhere our status is diminished, our expertise denied. No political party in Britain, socialist or otherwise, has coherently addressed our predicament. This is not just a problem of human rights denied: the right to full information about psychiatric treatment. It is also about the way in which a class of people have been invalidated, their creative potential ignored and their insight systematically disparaged. Mental health is a critical concern in post-industrial society. Yet the powerful in society by their actions suggest that those who have experienced the problems of retaining mental health at first hand have nothing valuable to contribute in this area. Even to the most reasonable, this hardly makes sense.

As a response to this situation a collective of present and former psychiatric patients have produced a film *We're not Mad ... We're Angry* to be shown on Channel 4 television. This is the first time a programme scripted and edited by the diagnosed mentally ill and entirely devoted to our viewpoint will be shown on the national network. The programme may not have balance. When you have been forced to stand on one leg for much of your life it is not always possible to retain

DOI: 10.4324/9781003636434-14

balance. But it does display an insight and commitment which as a special minority we are not often thought to possess. It was no easy thing to make this film. The material we have worked with has had and continues to have an emotional charge for each collective member. The arguments we construct are based on our own lives, not on statistics of deprivation. Whatever our awareness it is founded on experience.

We're not Mad ...We're Angry is the result of two years' work as a collective. Regardless of its qualities, its existence is proof of an alternative method to the psychiatric system. It is possible for a discredited group, that within psychiatric hospitals is encouraged to look to accredited expertise, to solve its problems, to look within itself, work together and be creative. The psychiatric model based on individual pathology, isolation and emotional life as an illness infecting the organism is not the only possibility.

It is perhaps appropriate that the genesis of this film has coincided with the startling growth of self-advocacy groups among users of psychiatric services in this country. It will no longer be possible to dismiss us as members of the 'Loony Left' and retain credibility. If we are members of the community, and such is the implication behind government and opposition policies, then we must be respected and valued as such. We are not seeking more treatments, better treatments, all the same treatments in smaller rooms with brighter wallpaper. What we seek is not 'treatment' but our own voice and a proper identity.

2.04

CARTOONS BY NIALL, 'MELVIN MENZ'

DOI: 10.4324/9781003636434-15

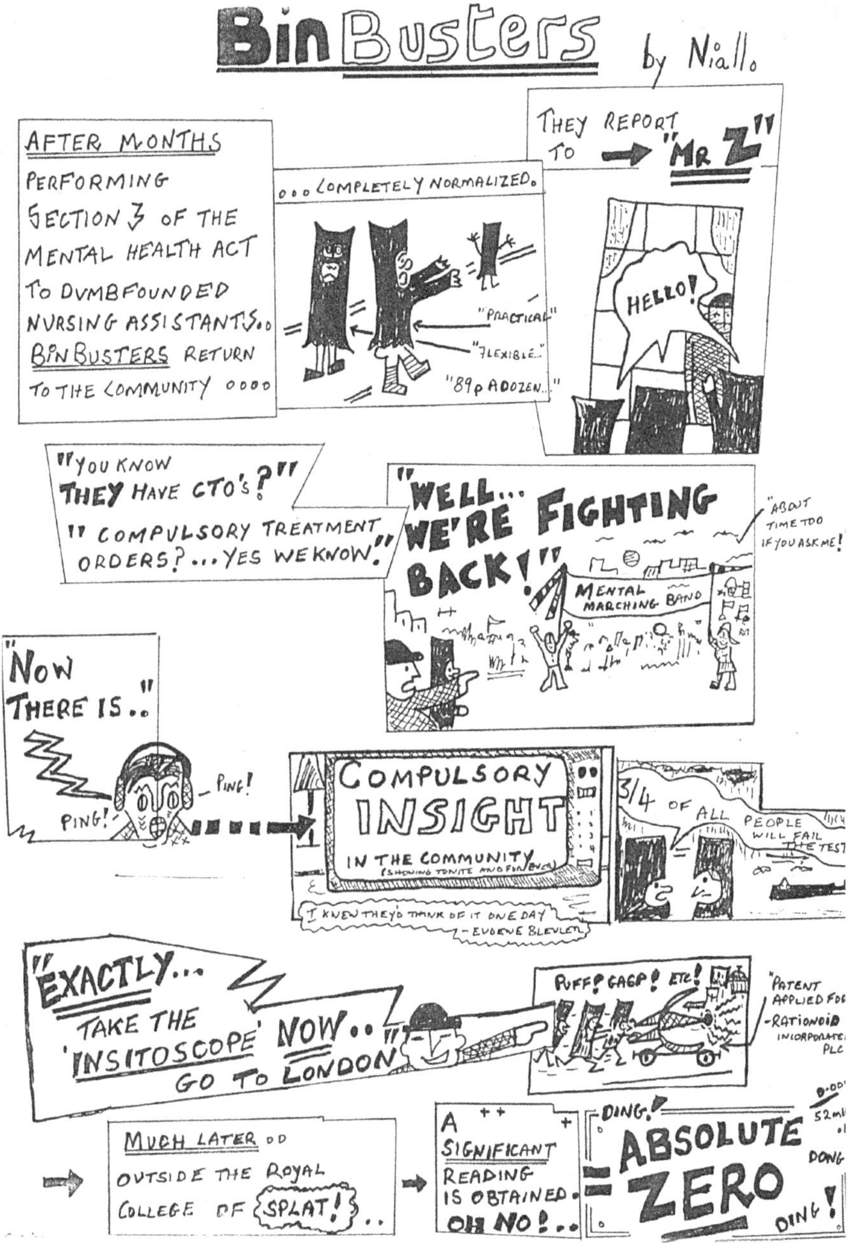
BinBusters
by Niall.
AFTER MONTHS PERFORMING SECTION 3 OF THE MENTAL HEALTH ACT TO DUMBFOUNDED NURSING ASSISTANTS.. BINBUSTERS RETURN TO THE COMMUNITY ....
... COMPLETELY NORMALIZED.
"PRACTICAL"
"FLEXIBLE..."
"89p A DOZEN..."
THEY REPORT TO "MR Z"
HELLO!
"YOU KNOW THEY HAVE CTO's?"
"COMPULSORY TREATMENT ORDERS?... YES WE KNOW."
"WELL... WE'RE FIGHTING BACK!"
MENTAL MARCHING BAND
"ABOUT TIME TOO IF YOU ASK ME!"
"NOW THERE IS.."
PING!
PING!
COMPULSORY INSIGHT IN THE COMMUNITY
(SHOWING TONITE AND FOREVER)
I KNEW THEY'D THINK OF IT ONE DAY - EUGENE BLEULER
3/4 OF ALL PEOPLE WILL FAIL THE TEST
"EXACTLY... TAKE THE 'INSITOSCOPE' NOW.." GO TO LONDON
PUFF! GASP! ETC!
"PATENT APPLIED FOR -RATIONOID INCORPORATED PLC
MUCH LATER .. OUTSIDE THE ROYAL COLLEGE OF SPLAT! ..
A SIGNIFICANT READING IS OBTAINED. OH NO! ..
DING!
= ABSOLUTE ZERO
DONG
DING!

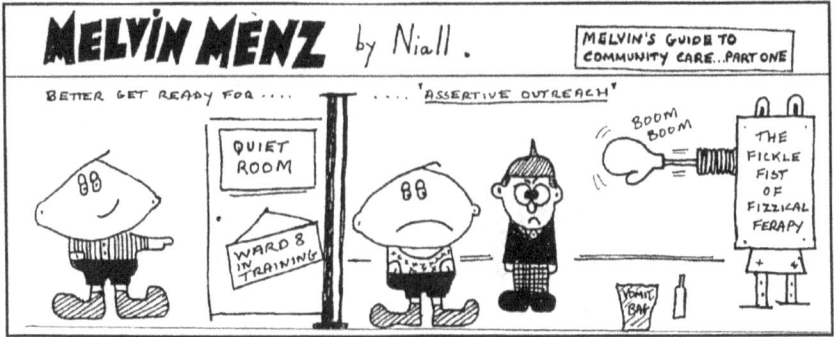

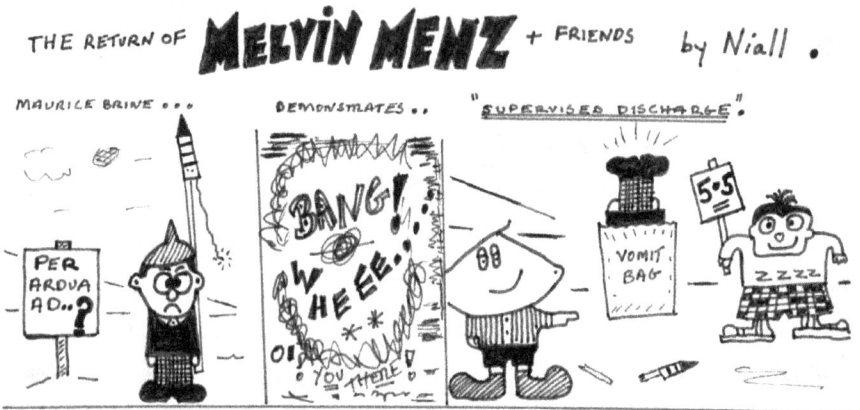

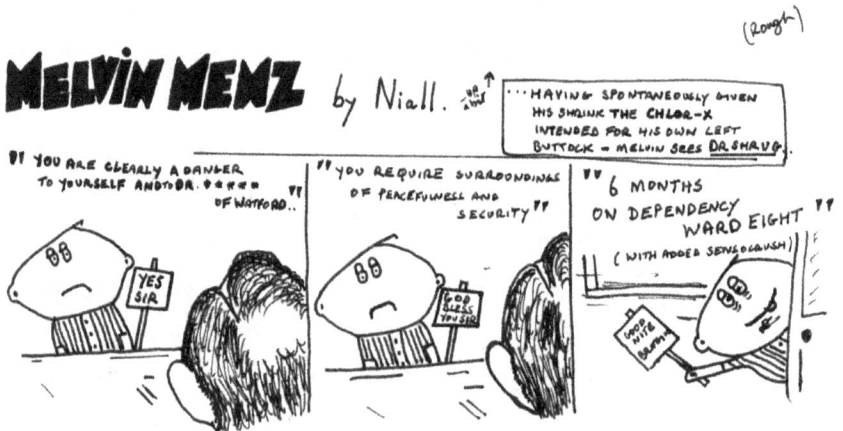

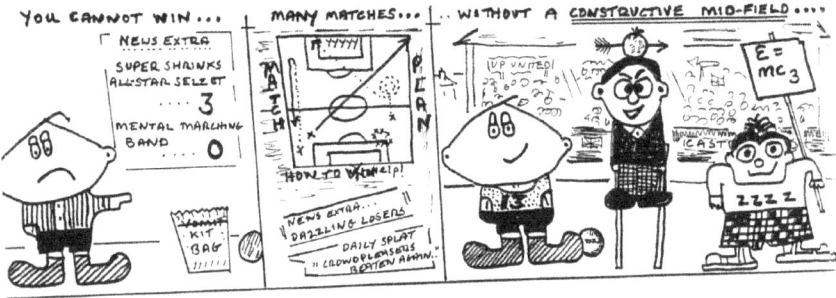

2.05

MADNESS CAFÉ [Abridged]

"The doctors want to see you Niall. I think you've got your marching orders". The staff nurse ushered me out of the day room. It was fifteen minutes to lunch. Turn right into the corridor and write again to the carpeted alcove. I took a breath and stepped into the consulting room. The entire care team seemed to be there, packed around the walls. The air vibrated with the sound of Intelligence Quotients waiting to perform. I sat down on the only chair left vacant. It was drawn out slightly towards the centre of the circle. The social worker's legs were well in evidence. It seemed just like the normal routine. Doctor Ingram, senior consultant psychiatrist at the hospital, looked in my direction and cleared his throat. It was like a great conductor tapping the rostrum with his baton.

"Mr. Parsifal, I believe the time has now come for us to part company. I think we must now discharge you. However bearing in mind your well-known reluctance to stay with us even as long as we thought advisable, this must be an occasion for some celebration".

Here he paused to collect the nods of his assembled team.

"So, what do you say to that?"

What do you say for seven months in the Bin? For being cut down alive from a dormitory pipe? For being locked away in a cell with only a slit in the door to let the light in? How do you assess five meals and fifteen games of ping pong every day of the week for 24 weeks?

"Thank you very much doctor Ingram", I said.

Leaving was the easy thing. I stood by the old gatehouse that wasn't a gatehouse anymore and checked my gear. Then it was off down the path to the bus stop. In town I had two cooked breakfasts in different cafés. Slow breakfasts with at least two cups of tea and no student nurse doing surreptitious observations from the next table. When I had my fill, I wandered around the town for the rest of the morning hoping I wouldn't run into anyone I knew. The local picture house had a spaghetti western on and I sat through its noise and violence twice to fill up the afternoon. Then I walked to the station and bought a single to London. I waited an hour and bought a six pack of beer from the shop. It was dark by then. By the time the train came in, I had almost changed my mind. I had a sudden flash of myself floating

 DOI: 10.4324/9781003636434-16

somewhere between the pavements of Piccadilly and the dark blue universe. But I climbed into a non-smoking carriage. The man with the red face caught sight of the six pack and made a space on his table.

I woke at Crewe and remembered I was mentally ill. Through the carriage window I watched them loading mailbags in the strange unhurried way that is a quality of stations in the middle of the night. My drinking partner of the early journey had gone. The seat across the table was empty. He had drunk the last can of my six pack and left the Glasgow evening paper spread out by the empties. I dozed from Crewe to the outskirts of London as the sky lightened. Just after Watford there was a squall of rain rattling all along the carriage windows. I could see milkmen in the street and little groups of people hurrying to the corner shops and the bus stops that reminded me of a picture I'd seen once in the north eastern gallery. Like all pictures, no matter how good they are you're always standing outside of them. Other passengers were moving now, checking their bags, combing their hair, and looking out of the windows to recognize how close they were to the terminus.

2.06

NUTTER's DIARY
[2 Sections, Abridged]

Section 1

Friday 3rd January

My name is Nutter. Alan Neill Nutter. Neill to my close friends, A.N. Nutter to the National Health Service and other official bodies. I'm a nutter. No messing. It's a bad joke but it's true. Like being a diagnosed manic depressive for fifteen years. Like missing relegation to schizophrenia by an absence of delusions and a change in the fashions. Like running around for fifteen years wondering what "with schizophrenic tendencies" means on an average morning.

I'm starting this journal for two main reasons. First, it's the season for it just now. Secondly, if I can behave as though my life is important to me, perhaps I'll keep myself together. *Per Ardua ad Astra* [a Latin phrase meaning, *Through Adversity to the Stars*, the official motto of the Royal Air Force] I do hope I stick around long enough to finish this journal.

Saturday 4th January

Today is my 32nd birthday. I breakfasted out at the Victory Café to celebrate. A good meal out and a football match in the afternoon is the best way to negotiate a January Saturday. Especially if you live alone.

Gino was behind the counter as usual. The way he moves around the cramped spaces, making tea, buttering rolls, and talking all the time would be magic on the edge of the penalty box.

"Same as usual?" he said, pouring out a tea.
"No, special day to-day Gino, I'll have tomatoes and a fried slice on top".
He smiled. "Building up something are we?"
"It's my birthday!"
"Sorry mate. Thought you might have a big date!"
"That's right. Match of the Day in colour!"
We both laughed. It's the same for him.

DOI: 10.4324/9781003636434-17

There are sixteen different words to express madness in the English language. Roughly. I thought up another two while I ate the food and drank two cups of tea. It didn't help very much but it was cheaper than a morning paper.

.... Rangers were beaten three-nil. The man next to me was arrested.

Section 2

Monday 5th January

Do the children know they are keeping me alive I wonder? Sometimes I think we are involved in a great conspiracy together and they've just never bothered to mention it. If I could work there for the rest of the year, I would be half-way home. You wanna bet on it!

Anand welcomed me by pissing all over the toilet floor. He stood slightly bewildered among the puddles at his feet and stuck his pinky in his mouth. I couldn't stop myself smiling. When he saw that, he came out with a huge grin and ran round in little circles. It took me fifteen minutes to clear the mess up and my cup of tea went cold before I could get back to the playroom. They never taught me about that in college.

At lunch Sarah and Stephanie said one of the lavatories was blocked and would I fix it. I said I didn't think that was appropriate conversation for meal times but they didn't laugh. I didn't see much of the children today in the end but I did discover why the toilet on our landing isn't working. When I got home, I fixed it.... Good-night.

Tuesday 6th January

No work to-day. ...In the end I did some work on a poem I hadn't been able to finish before. Surprisingly, it just flowed out and I felt good.

2.07

HOTEL GALACTICA [Abridged]

They've taken to painting seclusion rooms pink recently. The whole idea of seclusion has gone badly downhill since psychiatry got hold of it. I used to live in a secluded valley in Scotland, but it didn't have three walls and a locked and padded door. And it certainly wasn't painted pink. They paint hamburger bars in contrasting colours because they don't want people hanging around too long after they have finished eating. I guess it is this type of thinking behind pink seclusion rooms. You may be in there a long time, and there is nothing to do, so they paint it pink and hope you will remember the womb. It reminded me of the inside of a strawberry ice cream and I was the stupid ripple. Except it wasn't very funny. Except it wasn't funny at all.

I wouldn't wish to remember being in the seclusion room except that I cannot forget it. Not in Hotel Galactica nor in those other hotels further back. But the staff who run the Galactica seem to forget it pretty quick. In fact, they never even mentioned it after I came out. People keep on saying that these things never happen now and that the Hotel Galactica is an open place. But they do and it isn't. And if you look at the plans for the new range of hotels, you'll see plenty of them have a wee room they can do seclusion in. But they will not let you throw cushions in the corridor. Oh no. It will only do to put a loony's anger one place. And that is in his own arms. In a bare room. Alone.

Well, the next day they gave me a bath and walked me back to where I'd been the evening before. I was stood in the office and told I was on a section. They gave me the wrong Rights Leaflet so I pointed out the mistake and they gave me another one. What they were not able to give me were any shoes and socks, my own having been mysteriously detained in police custody the previous day. Instead, I was given a pair of Wellington boots two sizes too small and left to settle into the Galactica routine. When I reached the Day Room, I put the Wellington boots into the waste basket and rested my bare feet on the Rights Leaflet. I could see the next few days would be a piece of cake.

Micah came over later on and we sat and talked.

"You were a long way out last night", he said.
"I suppose so and they were giving me a good wee push too".
Micah nodded.

  DOI: 10.4324/9781003636434-18

"Doing the Magellan", he said and we both laughed.
I asked him what he was on at the moment.
"Melleril for men – lasts longer, cuts closer".
"And wrecks women too", I added. "Boom. Boom".

   We went on talking. Micah was under a new consultant. After a while, Erin came in and sat with us, listening but saying nothing. She had just come off "a special". And was in her nightclothes. Erin went way back to the days of insulin coma therapy and electroconvulsive therapy (ECT) without muscle relaxants. She was a bit of a legend to those who used the Galactica. In the end, Micah and I got talking about the old days, the multidisciplinary ward round psycho drama and the R.D. Laing word game. I began to feel safe again. We had begun the Professor Clare look-alike contest and were going for the triple bonus when Erin got up and walked out. "Don't mention Mr. Laing in the ward round, Micah", she shouted as she left. "He was a bampot – same as the rest of us".

2.08

'TYPING ERROR' (c1986)

When I apply for a job, I almost always get an interview. This is not because of any outstanding quality in my applications. Except that I am a man and therefore something of a curiosity. Even today, it is not usual that a man should earn a living caring for children under the age of five. Childcare, particularly for this age group, remains predominantly the concern of women. To some extent, and on more than one level, society actually considers male involvement to be abnormal. Men's prerogative to educate is reinforced, their capacity to care denied.

One of the reasons I began working with preschool children after my graduation was a belief that much school-based education is founded on an opposition and not a community of interests. Too much education is concerned with stuffing in rather than leading out. Training of the intellect sometimes seems to be incompatible with caring for the person. It is the same type of preconception as operates within the psychiatric system where emotional distress is seen as an illness and therefore inherently negative rather than as evidence of change which has the potential to be either good or bad. Such unchallenged assumptions condition many of our services.

In the beginning, the novelty of being a man working with under-fives was attractive. But there were disadvantages. When I began work the wages for nursery nursing were poor, based on the judgement that this was work for women who would soon be married, or for those, already married, who had an another, more substantial, wage packet in their household. Moreover, nursery nursing was not, and to a large extent still is not, recognized as a profession by many involved in childcare. It is impossible to avoid the impression that playing with young children to many people is not real work but what Dad does when he gets home from the office.

Many acquaintances were skeptical about my so-called career. Unusual certainly, but often also strange. At one nursery I discovered that a woman colleague assumed I was gay. Such a conclusion, although clearly an individual response, is to some extent a disturbing one in more general terms. The way we segregate supposedly male and female attributes, delineate them with ancient prejudices, and use them to value and devalue our qualities as human beings is not healthy. Not for us nor for those in our care.

 DOI: 10.4324/9781003636434-19

Having been invited for a job interview, there are two types of question that I have always encountered. The first concerns the special qualities that I believed a man could bring to a nursery. In broad terms, there are obvious advantages in having both men and women involved in childcare. The world is made up of women and men. A number of children may be brought up in single-parent families. For these and other reasons it seems obviously useful that children should have access to both adult sexes in early childhood. Even so, I would like to consider that being a man is merely a framework for whatever skills and experience I have acquired through study and practice and is not itself the summit of my contribution as a nursery worker.

The second area of questions always revolves, whether openly or by implication, around the issue of being a man entering an all-woman team. It is clear to me that a woman's idea of a team and a man's idea of a team are not entirely the same. I have encountered concern that I might take things over. While this is a valid issue in the context, it is also one which it is very difficult to address as an individual. I also know of at least one occasion when I have lost a chance of work because my potential superior did not feel she could comfortably give orders to a man. If you choose to enter an unfamiliar camp, you cannot avoid the doubtful reputation of foreigner.

Control and the fear of losing it is an inherent problem in all caring professions – childcare, education, psychiatry. Too often the professional workers' reluctance to being changed denies the chance of change in those they serve. In nursery nursing the adult's control can never be seriously challenged and true education can perish within omnipotence. In psychiatry the issues of control can appear so live that order is sanctified and the possibility that change and education might be essential elements of treatment is never adequately entertained. My own experience with pre-school children has made me a believer in care based on 'creative non-intervention'. In practice, this involves close observation and a sensitive attempt to make the child the real centre of concern. The power which the adult holds in transactions with young children, the power which the therapist and the psychiatrist holds over adults in distress, should be used with the utmost restraint. I do not believe education or care, and they are the same article, can exist without respect for the individual.

Typing the individual is endemic in modern western society. Indeed, it is difficult to see many professional and intellectual disciplines surviving without it. The major disadvantage inherent in typecasting is that it limits the full potential of social being and becomes a negative force. The widespread interest in those who go against typing is surely founded on the recognition of such restrictiveness. My own experiences as a nursery nurse and as a user of psychiatric services suggest that there are no reasons why a man cannot be creative and fulfilled working with young children, nor the so-called mentally-ill live dynamically within society. No reasons except that the implications may be awkward for the majority.

At one point, I was persuaded to give up working with children. Enlightened people told me that the mentally ill could not do such work. This is not true. The error of typing lies chiefly in the fact that it reasserts what we are not, while denying what we might become.

2.09

'LOSING & REGAINING CONTROL' (1986)

[An edited version of this chapter was subsequently published in 1989 as 'Peter Campbell's Story' in Anny Brackx & Catherine Grimshaw eds, Mental Health Care in Crisis, London: Pluto Press]

'On Tuesday I woke up an hour before my alarm clock and wrote half a poem before going to work. I did a full day and worked an hour and three-quarters unpaid overtime. The Christmas rush was coming and pressure was building up. On my way home a dosser approached me in Euston station. I bought him food and I spent two hours finding him somewhere for the night. By the time I reached home it was already late but I still managed to write three important letters before going to bed.'

'On Saturday I woke at dawn and left the house within half an hour. I felt tremendous. Things had finally slotted into place and I was going to convert the natives of the Upper Niger equipped only with inspiration and a portable gramophone. Two hours later I tried to cross the Broadway opposite Hammersmith Odeon with my eyes closed. I laid my possessions outside the door to the church by the flyover and built a diagrammatic Calvary on the path. By mid-morning I was in custody, picked up by the police while standing in a bus garage calling out about poisonous fumes in the earth. They locked me in a cell. I thought I was on the way down to Hades. Later they put me in a van and took me to a psychiatric hospital. I remember lying on the floor of a padded cell in my underclothes.'

The above scenario is a distillation of events from eighteen years as a user of psychiatric services. Whatever else it may reveal, I believe it illustrates a major feature of life for those diagnosed as mentally ill: loss of control. Loss of control, whether truly lost or merely removed by others, and the attempt to re-establish that control, have been central elements in my life since the age of eighteen. My argument is that the psychiatric system, as currently established, does too little to help

DOI: 10.4324/9781003636434-20

people retain control of their lives through periods of emotional distress and does far too much to frustrate their subsequent efforts to regain self-control. Whatever power I may now have over my life I have, to a large extent, won in spite of rather than because of psychiatry.

Before describing the specific processes of psychiatry as I have experienced them, I wish to make two general points which concern the context within which the system operates. The first relates to the medical model, or more accurately to the assertion that the phenomena psychiatry deals in should be seen in terms of 'illness'. Whether we accept this approach or not, there can be no question that it provides the current framework for society's view of the subject and that the psychiatric profession must take responsibility. Psychiatry would see itself as a servant of society. Yet it is naive to suppose that a profession with such individual and collective power does not form, as well as reflect, public attitudes. If we think of emotional distress as mental illness, it is psychiatry that has seduced us so. And the pre-eminence of this concept does affect individual autonomy. To live for eighteen years with a diagnosed mental illness is no incentive for a positive self-image. Illness is a one-way street, particularly when the experts toss the concept of cure out of the window and congratulate themselves on candour. The idea of illness, of illness that can never go away, is not a dynamic, liberating force. Illness creates victims. While we harbour thoughts of emotional distress as some kind of deadly plague, it is not unrealistic to expect that many so-called victims will enjoy limited, powerless and unfulfilling lives.

In the same way, the feeling that the diagnosed mentally ill don't know what they're talking about limits the scope of our lives. The concept of insight – perhaps lack of insight would be more appropriate from the psychiatric perspective – is one of the most powerful and insidious forces eroding our position as competent, creative individuals. If I am to be confined to a category of persons whose experience is devalued, status diminished, and rational evidence dismissed, simply because at a certain time or times I lost contact with the consensus of reality agreed on by my peers, then it is scarcely possible to expect that my control over my life will ever be less than severely circumscribed. If my experience is not valued, I cannot be whole.

It is currently quite unclear whether those who work in the psychiatric system place a high priority on maximising an individual's self-control during the process of breakdown. In this respect I find it significant that no psychiatric professional has ever advised me on how to cope with a breakdown beyond the blanket exhortation to keep on taking the drugs. My own experiences suggest that once I start to lose control again, I am expected to admit powerlessness, hand myself over to the experts, and count to 15,000. Such suspicions tend to be confirmed by the notably frosty reception of my own ideas about my treatment received from those who are attempting to process me back to an in-patient status. It is clear to me that it is inconvenient to have to consider the integrity of the new admission too carefully during absorption into the psychiatric system. It is clear to me that the system's needs dominate the individual's needs.

Whatever the intentions behind the system, the reality of current provision is clear enough. For those who experience severe mental distress there is only one destination – the psychiatric admission ward. Many of us – particularly those whose crisis occurs after the hours of sunset – will find the journey there extremely unpleasant. I have found GPs reluctant to visit me after dark, casualty departments where knowledge of psychiatry or psychiatric medications is peripheral, psychiatrists' secretaries who do their best to persuade you not to bother your doctor in times of acute need – in short, a network of provisions designed to make it difficult for me to receive the help I may need, and almost impossible to seek out the help I want.

If the admission ward met my needs, I would endure the process of admission and the absence of choice as necessary evils. But it is becoming clear that for myself and for many others the admission ward is in no way a satisfactory environment in which to recover mental health. The existing system is not sufficiently sophisticated, those who operate it not sensitive enough, for whatever reasons, to meet the real needs of the many individual people who are forced through it year after year.

In particular, I object to the way in which power is stripped from me, the way that I am approached not as an individual but as a manic depressive. It is not right that I should be casually dragged into unconsciousness on arrival in an admission ward. It is certainly wrong that I should receive such treatment regardless of whether I arrive handcuffed to a policeman or walk in of my own accord and calmly ask for help. On two occasions, I have been given so much medication that I fell asleep before admission formalities had even been completed. I have not yet been allowed to complete my own process of controlled breakdown without such ham-fisted interventions. While such practises remain common, it is not possible to claim that psychiatry respects individual integrity or is much concerned with self-education or change.

The psychiatric system is founded on inequality. By and large, the user is at the bottom of the pile. I have been on wards which could not have functioned without the active help of in-patients. Yet when conflicts arose, I have been told: 'what right have you to help with other patients? What would our union say?' I have met a few staff who clearly despise the 'mentally ill' and will openly abuse you. Their colleagues may agree in private that it is disgusting but they will always, in my experience, rally behind them when it matters. At times, it is hard work not to believe that we are a separate branch of humanity somewhere down there a bit.

Our unequal position is symbolised by the compulsory element in psychiatric care. I do not intend to argue either for or against the use of legal compulsion in treatment. But the fact of its existence has repercussions for all service users and these must be recognised. That an individual can be compelled to receive psychiatric treatment affects each in-patient, regardless of whether his stay is formal or informal. It is hardly possible to be unaware that you are being cared for within a legal framework which allows for treatment against your will. Moreover, it is difficult for most in-patients to long remain ignorant of the belief – whether based on fact or legend – that the threat of legal compulsion may be used to coerce individuals to accept particular treatments. Whatever the justification for compulsion in care, an inevitable result must be the diminution, whether physical or psychological, of the in-patient's control over his life. The implications of compulsion, the contradiction which may exist between the concept of compulsion and the concept of care, would seem to have some part in explaining why many psychiatric patients look back on their time in hospital as punishment.

Our self-image is further damaged by the limited extent to which we can participate in our own treatment and in that of our companions on the ward. While the resources of the medication trolley are over-used, the human resources of those living and working in the psychiatric unit are consistently under-used. I have been on wards where experienced in-patients have almost had to 'book' time to speak to nursing staff. I believe that many nurses whose prime impulse is to care for those in their charge are working in an environment which prevents them from exercising their most important human skills. Certainly, the potential of the in-patient to be a creative resource for the community of the ward is seldom realised. Patients do support one another. But staff attitudes to this are often ambiguous. I have seen the inside of numerous admission wards. With one notable exception, none of them have provided structures which actively encouraged patients to be involved in one another's care. Most ward meetings studiously avoid 'emotional' areas and do more to confirm the powerlessness of the patient within a bureaucratic system than to encourage participation. I have a distinct suspicion that mental health workers in general don't like us to get too uppity.

I believe such an atmosphere belittles the standing of the so-called mentally ill. We are encouraged to be victims, to look vertically to experts for the solutions to problems they have defined rather than to reach out for those around us who have a shared experience. We put down our positive capacities and assume instead the role of recipients of care. Our restricted role in our own treatment is of fundamental importance. The 'good' patient is usually the one who does what he is told. In one hospital a charge nurse told me that I would not be welcome on his ward in future because I complained about the quality of care. The implication that I should shut up and be grateful is disturbing. Participation, not passivity, should be the bottom line. I don't see conclusive evidence that the psychiatric profession always knows what it is doing. Simply to keep repeating their sagacity in a loud voice, does not mean that the experts are entering into dialogue.

At the crux of the dilemma is Freedom of Information. I don't believe a patient can be otherwise than powerless until he has reasonable access to information regarding his treatment. If there are choices of treatment, then the patient should be made aware of them. I do not find it proper to suggest ECT as a treatment without explaining its limitations and side effects, and those of the alternative treatments which are available. It is wrong to suggest, or to imply by omission, that there is only one course of action when it is not really so. I have vivid memories of the trouble mental health workers used to take in the 1970s to suggest that psychotherapy was not available, impractical, too expensive. I also remember how zealously staff guarded information about medication. Patients like myself, who knew something about the medications in the drug trolley, were treated with some suspicion. In general, I have found psychiatrists prefer to tell you the absolute minimum about the medications they have prescribed.

When I was put on Lithium Carbonate, I was told that it did not have side effects like other psychotropic drugs. It was four years before I was given a kidney and liver function test. Many of the side effects of lithium are precisely the same as psychotropic drugs – dryness of mouth and tremors for example – and there are significant possibilities of further effects from long-term use. All of this I discovered from my own researches. As a result, I was eventually able to weigh the pros and cons, and make my own decision to remain on lithium. But no thanks to the psychiatrists. The initial withholding of information, whatever it's motive, denied me one chance of exercising adult responsibility.

I am not aware of any conclusive statistics that revealing the true effects of drugs to patients ensures they stop taking them. Many of us stop taking psychotropic drugs because they do not do for us the things we have been promised they will do. Playing up the positive effects, and playing down the negative ones, is a recipe for trouble. The whole approach to medication in psychiatry seems to be tinged with the belief that the mentally ill are by definition incompetent, and unable to be adult, even when returned to the community. Information is not volunteered and even when asked for directly is given grudgingly and in adequate form. As a result of not being told the possible side effects of the depot injection Depixol when I returned to the community, I suffered sporadic side effects over a long period, culminating in my collapsing with paralysis of the lower limbs in a North London street. This frightening experience could have been easily avoided. But to do so, it would have been necessary for the system to recognise me as competent adult and a partner in change, not as a non-responsible recipient of care, biochemicals, and established wisdoms.

Every system has its faults. I would more easily tolerate the inequities of the process if the psychiatric system returned me bright eyed and bushy tailed among my contemporaries. But this it does not do. The percentage of re-admissions is high. Moreover, the diminished status we suffer while recovering from breakdown is not made right once we re-enter society. Discrimination affects us on major and minor levels, in personal and public areas. Discrimination in employment is standard. There are many with psychiatric records who are forced to rinse their talents down the sink and take jobs far beneath their capabilities. I find it humiliating to have to lie in order to be in with a chance of work. To be advised to lie, to choose to do so, and thereby admit a shame about my past which is not justified, and which I in no way really feel, has demeaned me more than any other single event of my life outside hospital. I want a chance to be what I am, and for that to be recognised as natural. Society is not only ignorant; it stuffs its ignorance down our throats as well.

My argument against the psychiatric system is not that it is uncaring. I have met individuals at all levels – nurse, social worker, psychiatrist – who were clearly caring people and have cared for me. But psychiatry must surely be more than custody and care. By approaching my situation in terms of illness, by regarding me primarily as the recipient of care and treatment, the system has consistently underestimated my capacity to change and ignored the potential it may contain to assist that change. My desire to win my own control of my breakdown process, and thereby to gain independence and integrity, has not only been ignored it has been thwarted. Throughout the last nineteen years, the major impression I have received is that I am a victim of something nasty, not quite understandable, that will never really go away and which should not be talked about too openly in the company of strangers. In short, I have been ill, am probably still considered to be ill, and am in some sense or other certainly handicapped.

I can find little evidence that psychiatry challenges the negative context within which the mentally ill live. By losing control, and having a nervous breakdown, I seemed to have entered a particular dimension of existence which is defined by the fact of its inhabitants' inability to have control of themselves, their environment, and their futures. The specific complaints I have made about the system's disempowering process are more worrying because they occur within an ethos that does not seem to challenge loss of power. Talk should be of creativity and change, not control and illness. Only then will the self-control I seek be a common object and not a by-product of protest.

2.10

SELF-ADVOCACY: WORKING TOGETHER FOR CHANGE (1990)

Presentation to MIND conference, October 10th 1990.

This presentation is given with memories of Charles Reed – a friend, founder member of *Survivors Speak Out*, and a fellow Scot – who died last Saturday morning.

I want to make it clear at the start that I'm not here presenting 'the users' perspective' or even a 'users' perspective'. I am making a personal contribution. I think this is important for two reasons. Firstly, I'm sceptical about the whole business of providing 'the users' perspective' at a range of events. What are the organisers' motives? What do they think they're going to get?

Sometimes I feel it's a bit like asking a Martian to say something startling about the back end of a train. Everyone applauds and says how wonderful. And after she's gone, they all say – but of course she doesn't know that the train is actually a mode of travel invented in the 1830s that revolutionised public transport and led to the rapid growth of Western-super-Mare and Brighton. Second, although I have been a user/recipient of mental health services for 23 years, and continue to use them, such use, such receipt, does not define my life. I hope, and believe certainly, that my life has been about more than consuming, or being consumed, by mental health services. I feel there is a real danger of people involved in mental health self-advocacy being caught in a psychiatric trap. How much do we restrict ourselves? How much do we restrict the view of others towards us by constant reference to the psychiatric system and our use of it?

Self-advocacy: the concept

I want to look now at self-advocacy – the concept. I have to say that I have some reservations about the term: self-advocacy. Does it make things clearer or more obscure? Every other time that we use the term, should we be spending three or ten or fifteen minutes explaining what we think it means?

It is worth remembering perhaps that there was a time *before* self-advocacy. What were we all doing then? What were they doing in the Mental Patients' Union in 1970? What were they doing in the 1860s in the Alleged Lunatics' Friends

DOI: 10.4324/9781003636434-21

Society? Self-advocacy is a phrase introduced from the outside which may have its own limitations. Personally, I've always thought the idea of self-advocating sounds a bit disgusting, like making yourself sick up on the day room carpet.

Part of the problem with the term is that it can seem contradictory. Advocacy, the root word, has a meaning of someone speaking and acting on behalf of another. If you then prefix it with 'self', I think you are bound to create confusion. In this whole field, I think there is a danger of band-wagoning. The old 'submarine in the cornflake packet routine', you know. Be the first in your gang to have all four colours: citizen advocacy, self-advocacy, professional advocacy, legal advocacy. And this ignores the fact that one of them may be a paddle steamer after all.

I think it is interesting that in mental health we had advocacy first and then, quite recently, self-advocacy. An illustration of the 'incompetent until proved otherwise' syndrome affecting the so-called mentally ill. As far as I'm concerned, self-advocacy is the vital element that holds the whole structure together. If people who can speak and act for themselves are being prevented from doing so, then creating specialised systems of advocacy is ultimately futile. Advocacy without self-advocacy does not make sense.

It is like keeping the baby and the bath, but providing talcum powder dispensers and not water. The baby will become very aware of all the skills it lacks, will take a good long time to get out the bath and put its clothes on, and will certainly never learn to splash.

As far as I'm concerned, self-advocacy in practise is about collective action for change. A lot of what I've been involved in is groups of people working together to define their *wants*, raising their self-confidence and their belief in the validity of their wants and then acting to secure them, What has been transforming for me in the last five or six years has been to be part of a collective action. No longer standing in the charge nurse's office, an isolated patient, asking for my rights. But working with friends, locally, nationally, internationally, to secure for ourselves what is necessary and rightful.

Levels of self-advocacy

There are a number of levels that word self-advocacy can operate: the level of the admission or long-stay ward or the day centre, the level of the district health authority planning systems, the level of national organisations or government department and many more.

But at the root is the individual. The critical need is for individuals to be involved in their own treatment and care. There is a fundamental need for information and choice to make such involvement real. The preliminary results of MIND's People First survey suggests recipients are not often able to exercise informed consent. Informed consent is absolutely basic and we must campaign together to secure it. In the same way we must use the Code of Practice to the 1983 Mental Health Act to ensure that the individual in the caring system receives the best quality care.

Despite the promised new world to be ushered in by the community care legislation, how much more power will the individual recipient actually have? Will there be a real say in the assessment and care/case management process? What is left now of the Disabled Person's Act?

Equally, until we have full information about the effects of medication – positive and negative – being made properly available to all, until proper systems are established to support those who wish to reduce or withdraw from their medications, how far can it be claimed that mental health services are offering choice in a meaningful sense?

Degrees of self-advocacy

As well as levels, there are degrees of self-advocacy. I believe self-advocacy should be about giving people power over their own lives, not just their lives within service systems, but their lives as a whole. In the field of mental health that involves a huge shift in attitudes, not just among mental health workers but in the community itself. Empowerment also means the acquisition, or re-acquisition, of a range of skills among this devalued group.

But how far down the road of empowerment are people currently prepared to go? Community care is littered with a series of newish concepts – self-advocacy, empowerment, user involvement, quality assurance, consumerism. Some of these ideas are not well defined. Although they all seem to be related, quite how they are related is not always clear or made clear. There is now a need for clarity. We need to discover whether what the government departments and other powerful groups of service providers are going on about is anything like the same as what user groups are working for. We cannot go on cosily assuming that we all have common concerns. Questionnaires devised and analysed by people who have probably never been on the receiving end is one thing. Proper consultation that works and, dare I say it, a direct say in running services, is quite another.

The 'user movement'

I want to say a few things about the user movement in this country. Not about its achievements – some of these will be covered in workshops later – but about the ways in which our contribution can be marginalised. One of these is representativeness. Who do you represent? You are not really representative…. Personally, I have always resisted the idea that the quality of your contribution, the quality of your evidence, depends on the number of people you represent. If a piece of nursing practise is bad, and devaluing, does it become less so because my organisation only has 52 members and even less so because they are all over 63 and come from Hendon?

Nevertheless, if representativeness is valued so highly, those who value it must give us the means to be representative and look to the representativeness of other groups in the game. To invent new criteria which cannot be met, simply because the folk on the ground floor have joined the party, is both wrong and hypocritical.

Second, articulateness. You're articulate, OK you are exceptions, you are not like the rest, you are frauds! Well, pancakes to that! Articulateness only separates because society has established, and still clings to, a stereotype of the so-called mentally ill as inarticulate and incompetent. Inarticulateness and a deaf audience are two different things. If, after years of not being listened to, of not being thought to have anything worthwhile to say, we achieve a voice, we must sustain it, dismiss such attacks, and give articulateness its proper value.

Another interesting example of the ways we are discounted is in the way a number of people who have been diagnosed 'schizophrenic' have criticised psychiatry on the media only to be met with a response 'Oh you were obviously wrongly diagnosed, you were never a schizophrenic really…!' BIG DEAL! It's like sitting on a box of soft fruit for three days, getting to your feet and saying, 'Oh I'm awfully sorry but you're a tomato not a plumb!' It's all very well as far as it goes, but the bruises stay just the same.

Finally, BEING A FACTION, a small politically motivated interest group. Well sure, we are a small young movement, and we are certainly motivated and active but how does that make us different, or inferior in class, to any other groups in the field? Carers' groups, professional associations, local and national MIND, the Royal College of Psychiatrists, user action groups, mental health self-advocacy groups, whatever you want to call them, are in essence no less, and no more, honourable than any of these.

But here I want to make a point, and I think it is a vital one. For behind this last criticism I believe there is an imputation that the user movement is not really interested in extending the value of recipients per se but only wants to push a party line.

This I would challenge most strongly. Although I, and many others active in the user movement, have clear and strongly held views on the psychiatric system and the status of its recipients in society, we are also aware about, and have personal experience of, the positive power of self-expression. And by that, I mean the ability to talk about our lives, and act in our lives, in the way we choose as individuals. Personally, I have not endured the seeming tyranny of the psychiatric worldview simply to impose another world system in its place. I believe that anyone who looks at the history of the user movement over the past five years will see that the attempt to privilege the voice of other recipients – regardless of what view is going to be expressed – has been genuine and strenuous. It is not impossible to hold strong views and to encourage structures that stimulate a diversity of expression.

The recipient view

Having said this, what is actually remarkable is how similar in broad terms are the concerns of people who receive mental health services. When people do self-advocate, to use that expression, what ends up on the carpet has a very 'samey' look. Talking to recipients from other countries soon leads to a shock of recognition of precisely shared problems and feelings. These shared perceptions, this solidarity, cannot be meaningless. Reading material from groups, here and abroad, leads to the same conclusion. There is too much, too much that is the same, to allow those in power to say we cannot act on this.

Mental health services are simply not good enough. You know it. We know it. When are we going to get something done about it?

A broader view

But this is not just about services. Self-advocacy should mean empowerment and empowerment does not stop at the clinic gate. It is my belief that services do not exist in a vacuum and that good quality services may not be enough in themselves. What we're talking about here is the misunderstanding and devaluing of a whole area of human experience, the existence of social, cultural, and moral trashcans into which large numbers of people are dumped for reasons that cannot withstand close scrutiny. What is needed is an extensive re-evaluation of that area of human experience we commonly characterise as mental illness. A re-evaluation guided by the insights of those whose experience we categorise in such a way.

It is significant that the user movement in this country is now not only working to transform mental health services but is also leading initiatives to reclaim areas of experience which have for years being totally the possession of medical and psychiatric perspectives. Last September, the first national conference on self-harm, involving people who self-harm and workers concerned with the issue, was entirely organised by members of the user movement. In the last year, work to open up an understanding of hearing voices which is not psychiatrically based, and to develop non-medical ways of coping, has been pioneered by members of the user movement and others.

I remember very clearly the occasion in the early 1970s when my consultant psychiatrist told me that what I thought, and felt, during so-called psychotic episodes was meaningless. That's about the same as telling an adolescent that love is a COLD TEABAG! STICK TO CHOCOLATE MILK! It simply doesn't ring true, and it rots the spirit. It is quite possible that understandings based on the shared perceptions of the so-called mentally ill may be helpful, and prevent the isolation and segregation of recipients. The exclusion we faced is based on the premise that we are different and alien in specific ways: we are dangerous, we are inarticulate, we are incompetent, we have no insight, no understanding. It is time we challenged these stereotypes directly and put them to the test.

Self advocacy: the broad sweep

One of the particular features of the experience of recipients is that we lose control of our lives or have that control removed from us. Self-advocacy is one way of regaining control, by working together to combat our powerlessness. To achieve this, we obviously need to be involved in our own care in treatment. We need to have a major say in the way the services that deliver care and treatment are planned, managed, and monitored. Beyond that, we need to have power to live in society and not be shackled down by discrimination over employment, by the difficulty in finding decent housing, by living on the borderlines of poverty. If we have all these things, we will be a long way down the road to self-control, to personal autonomy…. But, ultimately, we must realise that our powerlessness, our separation, our oppression if you like, is based on deeply rooted attitudes that contend that we are different, and negatively different, from our fellow human beings. Self-advocacy must challenge the unsatisfactory realities of our everyday lives. It must also attack the myths that sustain them.

Conclusion

I have spent a few years of my life in psychiatric asylums. There are many I know who have spent a good few more. But we're here now. In the body of society. This is where we belong. This is where we have always belonged. Here. Not there. In that other place, separated off like curdle.

It is possible that we shall all end up in that other place again sometime in the future. But that is not our place. That place was made for us. Out here is where we belong and that is where we're stopping. If the politicians and society don't like it, we have to teach them new social skills. No problem.

I'm grateful to have been part of the movement of psychiatric survivors in this country. I think it has done good things. I hope we get the chance to do a good bit more. Thank you.

2.11

'THE NEEDS OF PEOPLE IN CRISIS'

October 1990 was a bad month for me. In the course of a single week, I notched up my fourteenth and fifteenth admissions into a psychiatric institution. On this occasion, my crisis included spending eight hours in a prison cell awaiting assessment and delivery, discharging myself from the acute ward at 10:30 at night and conning my way back to central London on £2.50, another four hours in a prison cell, and a late evening admission into the safe haven of a seclusion room. In the end, I was placed on Section 3 of the Mental Health Act and discharged from hospital (still under section) in mid-November.

It is possible that such experiences are unusual in the lives of those who regularly receive the care and attention of mental health services. Certainly, not all my own admissions have been equally traumatic. Nevertheless, my encounter with acute services last autumn, an episode which in retrospect still seems overwhelmingly negative, has underlined my long-standing concern over the way services respond to people in crisis.

A feature of the 'user movement' in the last five years has been the consistency with which groups across the country have called for 24-hour crisis houses. At the very least, this reveals reservations about the destinations currently available to people at times of great distress. I share these reservations. For many people, myself included, the option of staying at home through a crisis is not appropriate. For us, the acute ward is the inevitable ending of our journey. The provision of crisis intervention services, the whole performance of involving approved social workers as the 'social perspective' in assessments for compulsory admission, can seem a bit meaningless if there are no alternative destinations in view.

Choice has become a critical issue because there is a feeling that existing services do not provide many of the fundamental wants of people in crisis. Groups of service users continue to ask for crisis provision that does not have a medical orientation. These requests must be addressed sooner or later. Either they are a relic of 'anti-psychiatry' and reveal an ideologically-based hatred of medication and the

[n/d, article for Helen Imam, *OpenMind, c 1990*]

   DOI: 10.4324/9781003636434-22

'medical model' or they are an indication that our systems of care are significantly failing to respond to human distress.

When I am in crisis, I almost always need a place of safety. But there are many views on what a safe place should be. A strong shack suitably fastened can be a place of safety. In certain circles, a prison cell can be defined as a place of safety, but the safety it provides is of a different order to that of a room filled with friends and loved ones. Making sure people are not a danger to themselves or others is one thing. Making them feel safe is something else. One of my criticisms of acute services is that they often promote a negative or neutral approach to the concept of safety.

The poverty of the acute ward environment can be very striking. This is not just a question of the physical surroundings. Although, when I was an in-patient last autumn, the day room windows let in huge draughts, there were not enough chairs in the dining room, not enough cutlery, no salt cellars. Nor is it about physical care. Although I believe there is some truth in the legend that the worst place in the world to have influenza is on an acute psychiatric ward. What is an issue for me, is the quality of communication between nursing staff and in-patient.

All too often, psychiatric nurses spend little time actually talking to in-patients. In acute wards I have known, there has frequently been a shortage of nurses. Those who are available in the communal areas seem too busy with close observation, escort work or other duties to be able to sit and talk. Meaningful contact is restricted to the last two and a half hours of the afternoon shift. A friend of mine has encountered a key-worker system where the staff stay in the office all day and you are granted a 20-minute interview with your special person. Whatever the reasons, the acute ward can become a sterile container where in-patients are fed, medicated and supervised while the nature and implications of their distress are not explored in human terms. Last autumn, while on the acute ward, I was demonstrably shaken by the deaths of two friends. At no point did I receive anything remotely like bereavement counselling. Observation without interaction, an approach psychiatric training still seems to encourage, can be a cold tool.

One symbol of the failure of psychiatric imagination are the practices that surround the policy of seclusion. There seems to be a fashion now for painting the walls of seclusion rooms pink and they don't seem to have that dry straw-like smell they had in the old days. But the essential quality of the experience remains much the same. For me, it is horrifying (literally) that at the deepest point of my distress I can be locked into a small room with only inanimate objects to relate to. Whatever the justifications for its use, seclusion should be recognized as being innately damaging and steps taken to minimize its impact. Over the years, I have never received support or counselling after periods of seclusion. Last autumn, my night in seclusion was treated as something unremarkable and never mentioned. Although the Code of Practice to the Mental Health Act lays down guidelines for the practice of seclusion, it seems to contain no recognition of the need to support people after the event. The abandonment and isolation of individuals in the pit of their crisis must be an event with psychological repercussions. Is it unreasonable that a failure to address this is seen as a failure to care?

Supporting people in crises is not easy. My concern is that we continue to develop systems and to promote disciplines that make sensitive and flexible support more difficult. Following my experiences last autumn, it has been suggested I should agree to compulsory admission on all future occasions, regardless of whether I want to be admitted or not. This would help the nursing staff give me a better quality of care. I find the implications of such a proposal rather ominous. While it is possible that I am becoming increasingly unmanageable as I grow older, it is just conceivable that my distress in crisis is related to the inappropriateness of the response. Making me less powerful in relation to the care givers may make the overall journey smoother. But it has a tenuous connection with the quality of care and leaves all the important questions unanswered. What is needed is a proper dialogue, not a reaffirmation of the status quo.

I am glad to be able to add a postscript to the above. Early in 1991, in conjunction with my advocate, I wrote a long letter of complaint to the hospital about my stay. As a result, we had a three and a half hour meeting with management representatives and my consultant psychiatrist. A programme of staff training conducted by service users has been agreed and will begin shortly. Perhaps dialogue is a possibility after all.

2.12

'SPIRITUAL CRISIS' (1993)

Published in *OpenMind* 61, February/March 1993.

Peter Campbell introduces a new series by exploring the spiritual dimension of mental health.

I am not an expert on religion. Like many other people, I have always been interested in spiritual matters. I usually watch '*Encounter*' and '*Everyman*' or '*Heart of the Matter*' on television at the weekend. My bookshelves contain paperback versions of the Dhammapada and the Tao Te Ching.

Organised religions have always made me uneasy, I am not a member of any church. My parents chose not to have me baptised. Nevertheless, at the age of seven I went to a school in the Scottish Highlands where religious instruction was of central importance, the Bible was studied and we learned passages from the New and Old Testament by heart. As a result, the stories of the Bible are clear and familiar to me. The imagery of both testaments is part of my consciousness.

I suppose I have a predisposition towards belief and frequently go into churches or other religious places to 'pray' (meditate/relax). I believe there are powers that we cannot see and fully understand – perhaps love, perhaps electromagnetism. Like many people, I am not indifferent to questions about the meaning of life.

At the same time, the course of my own life has been shaped, and to some extent diverted, from its expected direction by a number of occasions when I have gone through profound, vivid and disturbing interior experiences which might be considered to be spiritual crises. At these times – times of elation, exhaustion, anxiety, fear – I have lost firm contact with the reality accepted by those around me, have entered a space where other realities and other powers are more urgent, and have experienced the consequences.

Once, down Hammersmith Broadway, considering myself Christ-like, I laid out all my possessions by the west door of a church in a diagrammatic Calvary and was picked up for crying out in the street. Another time, more recently, I believed myself the cause and focus of an impending collision between the earth and the setting sun and was found mute and unmoving in the shade of a garden hedge on Dollis Hill, North West London.

DOI: 10.4324/9781003636434-23

Inevitably, my beliefs and actions at times like these led to a confirmed diagnosis of psychotic mental illness and all that follows from it. On more than one occasion, when I have been struggling to hold on to my humanity, uncertain whether I was good or evil, Christ-like or Satan, I have found myself locked up and abandoned in a cell, deprived of human contact, observed but not comforted.

Perhaps such desolation was particular to me. But crises like these, and the reactions they let loose, can move the individual a bit beyond fireside thoughts on the meaning of life. Fundamental questions arise. Who am I? What have I become? Am I truly human? For many people who have become 'mental patients', spirituality and spiritual understanding are vital concerns.

The relationship between madness, religion and medical science is complex and has a long history. The fact that in Western societies, we nowadays almost always talk of madness as 'mental illness' indicates the triumph of the medical (psychiatric) viewpoint that these human behaviours are predominantly to do with the mechanisms of the body and mind and not the workings of the spirit.

Nevertheless, if it sometimes seems to us that the religious/spiritual worldview currently exists within, and subordinate to, the medical/scientific worldview rather than vice versa, we should recognise that this is partly because we observe the situation only in Western cultures.

As Suman Fernando has said, '"Western scientific" medicine tends to exclude ethical and spiritual considerations but the indigenous medical traditions of Asia are different –and this applies, I think, to Indian, Chinese and Islamic traditions' [1].

In Asian cultures, religion and medicine, religion and psychology are not so sharply differentiated. The dichotomy between mind and body, a concept inherent in western thinking which can quickly lead to a separation of persons from their distress, is not so evident in non-Western cultures. While on the Indian subcontinent there has been a long tradition of the religious people also being the medical people, many survivors of the mental health system in the UK experience psychiatry as an inflexible discipline which cannot adopt an holistic approach and is suspicious or intolerant of discussions about belief and spirituality.

There has been much writing on the connection between religion and mental health. The introduction to a recent collection contained a list of nine or ten characteristics of religions that contribute to mental health, followed by a list of nine or ten more that were detrimental to it.

Many well-known systems of religious belief have been scrutinised to establish which aspects of them might avoid or encourage psychopathological behaviour. There have recently been attempts to create mental illness diagnostic categories to encompass the activities of various cults in America.

I do not know enough about world religions or concepts of mental health to comment on the value or danger of such work. Even so, as someone who sympathises with Thomas Szasz's contention that psychiatry is itself a belief-system amounting to a religion, I do find these researches have a peculiar fascination.

What concerns me most are the spiritual difficulties facing individuals who enter the mental health service system. How do they value their experiences in crises? How do they withstand the scrutiny of science? How do they locate themselves within a society that sees them as damaged human beings?

There are a number of possible responses to 'psychotic episodes'. One is to view them as aberrations without intrinsic value. This seems to be a common approach in psychiatry and is the one I have almost always encountered there. Although it is important to define the causes of crises, the contents are not important. They are not worth understanding or are not capable of being understood – 'like the workings of a steam engine whose pistons have fallen off', as a psychiatrist once put it to me. As a result, the main action that is necessary is to intervene, often in medical ways, to control the episodes and prevent them happening again.

While I do not deny the value of practical crisis prevention, I feel such an approach is destructive. It not only suggests to me that the contents of my crisis are dangerous and impenetrable, but also presses me to separate myself from them. This I cannot easily do. Nor, I suspect, can many who experience similar crises. They remain part of us. We want to incorporate our insights into our lives, not to bind them in protective wrapping and carry them around with us as hidden baggage.

I believe human beings are damaged by attempts to separate them from the contents of such crises, even if these experiences confuse and disrupt. Telling people that their perceptions in psychosis are meaningless, or have only negative value, places obstacles on the path to spiritual understanding. Ignoring the content altogether merely confirms our suspicions that we are already beyond the pale.

Approaches that place a high value on 'psychotic episodes' and seek to explore their significance in spiritual terms have a considerable history. Among personal accounts, John Perceval, a Victorian pioneer of the self-advocacy movement, left a detailed record of his exploration of his psychosis in the light of a Christian belief [2].

In more recent times, a number of psychiatrists have published reports of successful therapeutic approaches which rely on a sympathetic and valuing approach to psychosis. One, John Weir Perry, speaks of psychosis as a visionary state and argues that this process has similarities to 'the high arousal state that seers, prophets and messiahs customarily undergo on the way to formulating their newly conceived mythologies'[3].

I welcome such approaches. Not because I claim my experiences have any special significance for others, but because they give me the opportunity to place the contents of my crises within wider and more creative frameworks. It is no coincidence that user-led organisations are doing so much work to open out understandings of madness. Spiritual breathing space is fundamental to us. The Hearing Voices movement, which has developed in the Netherlands and the UK over the last ten years, is a notable example of a broad collaboration aimed at self-help and challenging traditional psychiatric responses to 'hallucinations'. Significantly, Hearing Voices groups are not replacing orthodoxy with orthodoxy. They include people who have never been caught up in the mental health system. They respect the contributions of diverse beliefs.

I want mental health services that are sympathetic to the spiritual dimension. I would certainly like mental health workers to address my experiences in crises. But I also want them to make connections with the more usual aspects of my spiritual life I mentioned earlier.

I have spoken with hospital chaplains of various denominations during 25 years of psychiatric admissions and I have found their perspectives increasingly valuable. Nevertheless, their contribution always seems marginal to the main purpose of psychiatric hospitals.

An institutional system that focuses on malfunction, spirituality, creativity and imagination can easily become separate speciality concerns, discussed at appointments with priests or in art therapy. People can be fragmented rather than being made whole.

Belief is a sensitive subject and I'm not arguing for the invasion of private worlds. But respecting something doesn't mean never touching it. I have twice run away from psychiatric hospitals and sought asylum in churches. On one occasion, I got involved in two or three days of religious conversations with a fellow patient which ended in his attempt to exorcise me in the ward quiet room. Nursing staff were aware of all these events. They even brought me back from one of the churches. Yet there was never any attempt to discover what all this meant for me. I often wonder if the rituals, the atmosphere, the day-to-day practice of in-patient care might not be very different if the caring team believed something spiritually important was going on.

The health system does change. Mental health services are already varied and the new arrangements for community care may encourage greater variety. Alternative and complementary approaches are now more common. It is more likely that people with a diagnosis of psychotic illness will receive talking therapies. Perhaps the huge investment in technological solutions will never completely displace spiritual healing and dialogues on the meaning of madness. But we still live in a society that is suspicious of belief and connects unconventional belief to madness. Service users can end up in a trap, silenced by the prejudices of fellow citizens, their integrity doubted both by traditional psychiatry and major religions.

During my first stay in an acute ward, I read *The Politics of Experience and the Bird of Paradise* by R.D. Laing [4]. I didn't understand large parts of it. I still don't. But he did let me see that what I was going through could be part of a spiritual process and that the journey might be worthwhile. It has been something to hold onto. Psychiatry, and the society it serves, has rarely been so generous. That is one reason I call myself a mental health system survivor.

Peter Campbell is a founder member of *Survivors Speak Out*, the self-advocacy network.

1 Suman Fernando in *Concepts of Mental Health in the Asian Community* (Confederation of Indian Organizations, 1991).
2 See Dr Edward M. Podvoll, *The Seduction of Madness: A Revolutionary Approach to Recovery at Home* (Century, 1991).
3 See John Weir Perry, *The Far Side of Madness* (Prentice Hall, 1974); *The Roots of Renewal in Myth and Madness* (Jossey-Bass Publishers, 1976). John W. Perry quote is from 'Psychosis as Visionary State in Methods of Treatment in Analytical Psychology' (International Congress of the International Association for Analytical Psychology, Fellbach, 1980).
4 R.D. Laing, *The Politics of Experience and the Bird of Paradise* (Penguin, 1967).

2.13

"THE LAST COMMUNICATION"

I was two days into a crisis. I thought the house was surrounded by IRA snipers and that I would be shot if I went outside. I was marching up and down the staircase defending the property someone had called the crisis intervention team they came knocking on the door I shouted at them to go away they refused I opened the door I thought I was going to be shot at I told the social worker to stand back he refused I slapped him across the face with the palm of my hand the police were there I was interviewed by the crisis team and taken off to the asylum.

It was a few years later in the same asylum. Two evenings previously I had discharged myself after a couple of days inside. I hadn't felt safe. I lost my house keys and was picked up by the police. I spent a good few hours in a cell awaiting assessment. Now I was back on the ward for a night-time readmission. I was very distressed and angry. I think they felt they could not cope just then. After a while, one male nurse grabbed me. He hit me behind the ear with a bunch of keys, then he and the other male nurse took me into the nursing office and restrained me on the floor for some minutes. They were talking to me, they were not trying to comfort me. Later on, I was put in a car and taken to another ward. They marched me to a seclusion room, locked me in and left me there for the night.

These are two violent incidents from my own life within the mental health system. They do not represent the only violence I have experienced or witnessed nor are they particularly newsworthy. Nevertheless, they are perhaps more characteristic of the problems most people will encounter in services than the dramatic incidents of extreme violence that have been given such attention by the national media recently. While the events surrounding the deaths of Jonathan Zito, Georgina Robinson, and Orville Blackwood are tragic and scandalous, violence in mental health services often has a more humdrum and insidious aspect.

I believe much of the current debate is unhelpful because it focuses on a small portion in a rather wide range of expressions of anger and violence and distorts the real situation even within this narrower spectrum. A tenth of psychiatric in-patients

[an article for *OpenMind*, 1993]

DOI: 10.4324/9781003636434-24

commit violent assaults on NHS staff. The rate of committal for manslaughter by mentally disordered people has remained constant throughout this century despite the belief that homicide is increasing as a result of community care [1].

At the same time, it is clear that health services are often not safe places. Harassment, bullying, verbal abuse, threats are a feature of most care systems. The results of a *Nursing Times* survey 1993 into sexual harassment at work, or in work related contexts, showed that 97% of women nurses who responded had experienced sexual harassment. Although clients were the largest single source of harassment at 30%, the majority of harassments came from other categories [2].

Women recipients of mental health services are particularly vulnerable. Many have entered psychiatric units as a result of violence they have endured in their lives. They will often fail to find a safe place there. I know a number of women who have been sexually harassed as in-patients in recent years. They all speak about the difficulty they faced in being taken seriously and how little seemed to be done when they were believed. But it is not just women who feel unsafe. In many psychiatric wards, where people feel powerless fearful and confused and staff are unwilling or unable to make sustained sympathetic contact, safety may have a negative rather than a positive quality.

Michael has been surviving in the mental health system since the mid-1960s. He believes "you can only feel safe when you have the key to the door". He feels there has always been a strong element of fear within institutional care. Fear of the unknown and hierarchy can create an atmosphere stimulating violence. Although "primary violence" is less likely now, violence has been "intellectualised". He talks about receiving "boot therapy" from a charge nurse in the old days – a mixture of kindness, frustration, and violence you might expect from an older brother. Such an approach may no longer be tolerable, but mutual aggression remains reinforced by imbalances of power and the fact that "staff are paid to stay in control". Behind everything lies "the great misunderstanding", the conflict of perception about what is going on when people are in distress.

Melanie's son is diagnosed as mentally ill and has acted violently on occasions. He has been in a secure unit and was assessed for transfer to a special hospital. She does not feel violence has been a prominent concern for her. Nevertheless, she's keenly aware that services can be psychologically violent, "both aggressively in what they do and passively in what they neglect to do". She feels people's basic needs are often not met. She knows her son perceived every injection as an act of violence and felt his confidence and personality was being "stolen away".

Melanie views the affirmation of value and identity as vital to recovery. Therefore, "we need to be very sensitive to violence but must ensure that a full range of feelings are accepted". Both she and Michael spoke about manipulation and frustration, the pervasive boredom and barrenness of hospital life and the need to open up new dialogues. "The staff are angry and never allowed to show it either", Melanie said.

Duncan has been a residential social worker and a probation officer. He now works for a local MIND association whose services include housing and drop-in clubs. Although he acknowledges the risk of violence in community services, he doesn't feel it is an unacceptable one. Violent incidents at the drop-ins are "not uncommon". "The mixture of clients, and not knowing enough about people", makes it difficult to avoid incidents. But there have never been so many that people stopped coming. There are guidelines for workers and volunteers on who should deal with potential violence, what to do, and how to extricate yourself from difficult situations. In one drop-in, the users' group is developing guidelines on acceptable behaviour. Whatever the problems, Duncan feels it is vital to provide clubs for people who will not use more selective services.

Following a major incident in one of their houses, the MIND association is quite cautious about establishing new services. Duncan thinks this has been helpful, both by encouraging closer scrutiny of premises design, and the use of security-aids like cordless telephones, and by enabling staff to examine their own jobs, and press for better conditions and training. Duncan still believes good information, adequate staffing, and systems of care can make community care effective, if not risk-free.

The main problem with violence in mental health services does not appear to be that we know too little about it. In recent months, *Nursing Times* and *Community Care* magazines have been full of articles on coping with violence and aggression. The predicament of women and of Afro Caribbean men has been featured in campaigns over the last five years. Nor is it true that nothing is being done. Guidelines and policies are being written. There is innovative work like developing de-escalation models of control and restraint and the anger management groups run at Reaside Regional Secure Unit [3].

But is the full range of problems being considered? If people's violence is not persistent or particularly disruptive, how carefully will it be addressed? In our concern about violent assaults, are we overlooking the impact of therapeutic aggression? We should also be aware of who is being involved in the discussion. Melanie felt she had been manipulated to control her son's behaviour. She also felt "shut out, not heard". Michael is still not always sure whose side the staff are on. Unless we talk across these boundaries, we are simply building up more frustration.

No mental health worker has ever spoken to me about the violence in which I have been involved. At the time I struck the social worker, I was working with preschool children and found the personal implications hard to resolve. My night in solitary confinement was never remarked upon.

Michael sees violence as "the last communication". It may often happen when more constructive interactions have broken down. Better guidelines, better staff levels, and better environments will certainly help. But while society continues to see our crises as signs of mental illness, and thus fundamentally dangerous and incommunicable, our journeys through distress may continue to be unnecessarily lonely and violent.

References

1. Elaine Murphy, 'Could do it better', *Care Weekly,* 18 November 1993.
2. *Nursing Times,* 24 February, 1993.
3. Reaside Regional Secure Unit, anger management and de-escalation model, *Nursing Times,* Mental Health Supplement, 8 February 1995.

2.14

'VALUING PSYCHOSIS – A PERSONAL VIEW' BY PETER CAMPBELL

I have changed the title of this presentation from the one that appears in your conference programme. The title I am working to is: *Valuing Psychosis – a personal view*. In the time allotted I want to look at some of the challenges facing people who want to place a value on their so-called psychosis and at the wider problem of valuing that confronts those who live with what society chooses to call mental illness and I would rather call distress or madness. I feel my contribution today is a starting point for discussion rather than anything definitive.

To start I want to be clear that, for me, valuing psychosis is actually valuing psychotics. Perhaps this has something to do with the fact that I am standing before you as a very well documented psychotic. I know there are always attempts to separate the psychosis from the person. 'Och, it's not the *real* Peter' is a phrase that has echoed down my adulthood, with varying accents and additions from friends, relatives, nurses, social workers and psychiatrists. While I can understand the reasoning, and acknowledge the good intentions, that sometimes lie behind this chorus, it doesn't work for me. Nor for many of us. I may not enjoy psychosis, seek it out or feel it is one of my most useful capacities. But is undoubtedly an aspect of the real me. Excision of it would be my extermination. The lives of people who experience psychotic episodes are always to do with a great deal more than psychosis. This is true even for those who have persistent perceptions and behaviours that experts will define as symptoms of psychosis. But our lives, our past, our future, our destinies can easily be dominated by our capacity for psychosis and, in particular, by the predominant social responses to it. In this predicament, my bias is towards integration and reconciliation rather than separation and denial. I also feel that psychosis is about people rather than about phenomena.

The only cogent reason for my giving a talk today is that I am a psychotic and have spent much time in the last 25 years in the company of psychotics. I am

Prepared for the 2nd International Conference on Psychosis at the University of Essex, 22–23 September 1994

DOI: 10.4324/9781003636434-25

not a researcher and I am not a scientist – what academic training I have is as a medieval historian. Nor am I an expert – I don't take the position that that having had personal experience of psychosis makes me an expert on it. (Although as a result of psychiatrists' continuing uninterest, I do currently claim to be the only expert on the content of my own psychotic episodes.) My qualification and my bias is that I'm someone who has been admitted onto the psychiatric acute ward on sixteen occasions over the years, fifteen of which have been deemed to be as a result of a major psychotic illness, and that I have spent a lot of time, indeed an increasing amount of time, considering what the hell has been going on here…. In this respect, I do not think I'm very different from any other psychotic I've ever met. We're all wondering what has hit us. I cannot claim to have reached any startling conclusions. All I can hope to share is my/our predicament as I see it and to indicate something of the struggle I and others have had to find a new value to our lives.

As soon as I began preparing this presentation, I realized how rarely I have ever spoken in public about the content of my psychotic episodes. Nor have I heard many mental health system survivors speaking on these topics. As someone who has frequently been invited to speak at conferences, seminars and meetings as a mental health service user, I suppose I have had more opportunities than most. Yet I have not taken the chance to speak on this subject. I believe most survivor-activists in this country have been similarly reticent. Why has this happened?

The simplest answer is that we are usually not asked to talk about psychosis. Most of those who are increasingly handing out the invitations to involvement are interested in us as consumers, not as psychotics. They want to hear us talking more as users of services than as people with life-stories. The contents of psychosis, of psychotic episodes, are in some sense 'dirty' material – too potent, too personal, too disturbing to the framework of the discourse within which mental health services are planned and provided. There are businesses to be run. What is wanted is rational participation with just enough personal anecdote to spice the dressing.

And such an approach is understandable to an extent. Talking about psychosis may be very personal and disturbing. Airing such 'dirty' stuff in public can have unpredictable effects. I have always felt that the main problem I and other psychotics face is the belief that we are somehow quite substantially different to other sorts of people. When I have written and performed poetry, I have largely avoided attempts to describe my interior world during psychotic episodes. I have always believed such accounts would be likely to be viewed as essentially alien, freakish, other-worldly by most audiences, however sympathetic, and would ultimately do more to reinforce rather than erode underlying barriers. At the same time, I've also felt that most of the famous personal accounts of psychosis that I've read, whether in fictional or non-fictional writing, have failed to capture the quality of my own experiences and have seemed unconvincing and flat. This is probably inevitable. When you can be the director of your own science-fiction spectacular, Dr Who is always likely to seem less than satisfactory.

Coming out of silence

I believe two important considerations arrive at this point. The first concerns the way in which we conduct our public talking, writing and thinking about the content of psychosis. If we want to open up the possibilities of personal and social re-evaluation, what sort of languages should we be encouraging? Society has developed particular artistic conventions for dealing with its fascination for psychosis/madness. Are these any more or less helpful than the general mass-media enhanced stereotypes of the so-called mentally ill as a whole? Where can the personal accounts of psychotics fit when confronted by the manipulated chorus of public prejudice and titillation on the one hand and the monologue of inscrutable professional expertise on the other?

The second and perhaps most fundamental question is – how can anyone who experiences, or has experienced, psychosis be in a position to evaluate or re-value this capacity of their lives as a result of it when the experience itself remains such as taboo area? If no one will talk sensibly or sensitively to you about psychotic perceptions, how can you make liveable judgements? If talking about your dreams was beyond the pale, how many people would have handed back their member-ship years ago? Denying open discussion of profound and confusing aspects of the human psyche does not make them go away. But it can madden significant numbers of us generation after generation. If my contribution today has any one message, it is this: let's start working to cut out the silence.

I have two very strong memories from my first psychiatric admission 27 years ago – the only admission I've had that was deemed at the time not to be an outbreak of psychotic illness. I had just arrived at an English university from Scotland and within four days had panicked –the experts chose to call it 'acute anxiety neurosis'. I was admitted to an annex of a major hospital and given barbiturates prior to a deci-sion to send me back to Scotland, to a lunatic asylum nearer my family. Just before I travelled back, my leg and arm joints seized up. They discovered I was allergic to the medication. As a result, I was carried out on a stretcher, taken down to London by ambulance and put on the sleeper train north. What I remember most vividly during all this was the complete feeling of failure that enveloped me. This was an event not of medical significance but of spiritual and moral significance. Although I was not going to die, I believed, and to an extent believed correctly, that I was finished as a person. What this breakdown meant was not the start of a process of illness but the collapse of a personal and positive world framework and the entry, or at least the first steps of an entry, into a completely different and negatively ori-ented world. In a sense I had already crossed one boundary over which there is no return – I had become one of those 'loonies from Murthly' that my brothers and I joked about in childhood. Within four years, two more admissions during which I began to experience what the experts call psychotic symptoms and lost contact with the expectations of my peers, confirmed my identity as one of the mentally ill/the mad – a new and worse version of what I once thought I had been or would become.

So that is my first memory – of a profound moral failure, of a descent into a lower order. Feelings that still remain. Feelings that psychiatrists – healers of the soul – have made scarcely any attempt to acknowledge, let alone address, over the last 27 years. But my other memory is a more positive one. While I was recovering at Royal Dundee Liff Hospital and trying to make sense of what had happened – I was eighteen and I suppose that asylum was my first experience of adult life – I was fortunate enough to buy a copy of R.D. Laing's *The Politics of Experience and the Birds of Paradise.* While I cannot say that I fully understood (then or now) much in Laing's book, it does contain a description of a journey into and through psychosis that I found, and still find, extremely useful. R.D. Laing's suggestion that this process could perhaps be lived through without medical interventions, and could perhaps have meaning and be valuable in an individual's overall journey through life, was very important to me at the time – right at the start of my own career in the mental health system. I still believe it is a valuable contribution towards a psychotic's self-understanding, and self-acceptance, and is one that I have found worthwhile holding onto – perhaps I should say struggling to hold on to – throughout my years as a recipient of psychiatric interventions. I know it is now unfashionable to give any credit to R.D. Laing. Indeed, I witnessed an eminent psychiatrist indulging in a quite gratuitous attack on R.D. Laing at a conference not so long ago and I understand this has not been so unusual in certain quarters in the last few years. I never met R.D. Laing and I'm neither a disciple nor an advocate of his work as a whole. But he was certainly the first, and remains one of the relatively few, psychiatrists I have encountered who was prepared to assert openly that my psychosis might actually be worth something. I'm indebted to him for that.

Those two personal memories encapsulate something of the predicament that confronts most people who end up with a diagnosis of psychotic illness. Whatever our backgrounds, our education, our achievements beforehand, it is clear to us that something of major negative significance has happened in our lives. In the ensuing years, the questions that arise are not simply about, how do I stay well? How do I hold down a job, a flat, a social circle? How do I get up in the morning? But, also, to do with who exactly am I now? What have I become? What do these unusual perceptions mean for me? What quality of a person am I?

The way that individuals answer these questions or seek to answer them will always depend to some extent on the impact of so-called mental illness on their lives. The same will be true of symptoms of psychosis or psychotic episodes. My personal capacity for psychotic perceptions and behaviour is an episodic one. For many months I will not display thoughts, feelings or perceptions which anyone – least of all myself with my highly conditioned sensitivity to these issues – would class as unusual. Then over a period of ten days or a week, I will experience psychotic symptoms to a fairly intense degree before entering into another long period without them. Clearly, the difficulties I encounter, including the problems around placing a value on my thoughts, feelings, perceptions and behaviours, may be significantly different from someone who is every day, or for long periods of time, seeing and hearing things other people do not see or hear, or experiencing colours with greater intensity and increased significance or feeling the shape and texture of their skin changing. And so on. I am not trying here to make any claims of categorization around degrees of difficulty in valuing different types of experience, although my own observations suggest that people whose unusual thoughts, feelings, perceptions and behaviours are more continuous are likely to experience more distress. I have found valuing my psychotic episodes difficult enough as it is. Perhaps the fact that they are so intermittent and so well-defined has created problems of its own – certainly it seems to have given outsiders, including mental health workers, the encouragement to advise me to dismiss them altogether.

I can only theorize about the problems people with a diagnosis of psychotic illness face in giving a value to their psychosis. I am not aware that anyone has ever asked a group of such people what they feel the problems are. Perhaps it is not considered a worthwhile, or relevant, question. Perhaps I have not read the reports. All that I can present here are my own thought and opinions on the subject, the evidence of friends and fellow survivors of the mental health system (much of which is generally supportive of my own experience), and some hunches based on what I have read and assimilated about the world of psychiatry over the years since I first qualified for its care and scrutiny.

Obstacles to finding value for psychosis

Making use of the above (admittedly partial) evidence, my impression is that the major obstacle to individuals finding their own value for psychosis is psychiatry itself. When I say psychiatry, I suppose I mean more exactly NHS psychiatry as it has developed in the United Kingdom since the end of World War II – but I don't feel that is substantially different from psychiatry in any Western industrialized nation during the same period. I don't suppose that many of you who have followed me this far will be surprised at this impression. It is thought to be a characteristic of activists in the mental health field, particularly survivor-activists, to blame everything on psychiatry. Even so, whether the revelation is original or not, I have to underline that for myself, and many like me, the greatest obstacle to individual valuing of our experience is an approach asserting that this experience is intrinsically negative, essentially meaningless, something connected fundamentally to disease (but we cannot tell you exactly how and certainly cannot cure it), and something that we can, and will, suppress and/or remove from you, regardless of your views about it (oh, and incidentally we have legal sanctions to validate our way of looking at things). This kind of approach presents huge obstacles, one might almost say insuperable obstacles, to any autonomous or creative process of valuation. This, I would contend, is exactly what psychiatry accomplishes.

I believe there is a net of interconnected approaches and attitudes that capture and disable people here. It may not be particularly useful to separate them out and look at them individually. Nevertheless, as this is a personal view, I am going to take the opportunity of identifying what I find most damaging and debilitating about the psychiatric response to my psychosis, perhaps it will strike some chords in you.

In some ways, I feel I could handle my predicament better if psychiatry and psychiatrists declared to me openly: psychosis is negative, bad, evil. The perceptions within psychosis are harmful and must be shunned. The behaviours/actions they lead to are perilous, self-destructive and not acceptable to those you live among. Although I would disagree with large parts of such a proposition, it would at least be something I could engage with and challenge. The real difficulty for me has always been that while it is clear that society assumes that psychosis is a predominantly 'bad thing' and psychiatrists, as the agents of accepted expertise on psychosis that I've most frequently met, seem to support such an assumption, they don't really want to talk about it further. The way in which such reluctance has always been conveyed to me over the last quarter of a century and more is: the contents of your psychosis are meaningless. And there we have what I perceive to be the perfect double-whammy for nullifying an individual's experience and holding it in a state of indefinite suspension: a supposition of intrinsic but ill-defined negativity and a categoric repetition of meaninglessness.

It has always struck me as ironic that psychiatry should place so much store by the concept of 'insight' when it has such a narrow view of what insight could mean and is conspicuously not very interested in looking into various aspects of my or other psychotics' lives. Like so many other terms used in mental health care and treatment, the psychiatric concept of insight seems to be a largely negative one – lack of insight seems to be what psychiatrists are most interested in and perhaps that is because lack of insight among their clients is one of the main justifications for the power they can wield over us. But in my experience, the psychiatric conception of insight is also of an essentially static and medical nature. Some people have it and some people don't (I remember a staff nurse at Murray Royal Hospital in Perth during my second admission trying to comfort me by saying: 'You'll be alright son, you're got insight', like a benediction). Some people may lose insight during an outbreak of illness/psychosis but regain it when the illness is in remission. The idea that insight could be something that people might acquire by enquiry and by learning about themselves, particularly if that means asking questions about the nature and significance of a person's inner world during psychosis, or indeed at most other times, does not appear to be a prominent feature of the psychiatric enterprise. I once asked an eminent psychiatrist and social anthropologist what he thought the psychiatric concept of insight really amounted to. He replied: 'Agreeing with the consultant's plan for treatment....'

So, how has psychiatrists' assertion that the contents of psychosis are meaningless affected me? (I'm concentrating on psychiatrists here, because I feel their reactions on this topic have had a particular impact on me. I also feel the lack of sensitivity to psychosis among other mental health workers is important. I hope this will become clear in a minute.) Well, on one level I suppose I soon learned to lower my expectations about what aspects of my person and my life, psychiatry and psychiatrists were actually interested in. Like many other people who receive care and treatment from psychiatrists, I learned that there were certain questions psychiatrists asked which were not really open questions. They were asked questions to elicit set responses, not to open up a discussion, not to begin an exploration or enter into a dialogue. For example, it doesn't take any psychotic too long to work out what the question 'Do you hear voices?' is likely to be leading or not leading to. This is the start of a heavily scripted conversation, not a free and creative interaction. The destination of the enquiry has been largely pre-determined.

At the same time, I soon accepted that there were certain things I would not bring to the surface when in psychiatric care, certain aspects of myself that I would not try to share. In retrospect, I find it interesting to note some of the questions I have never been asked while an in-patient in a psychiatric institution. For example: 'Do you believe in God?', 'What do you believe in?', 'How do you feel about being "mentally ill"?', 'What's it like to live with a diagnosis of psychotic illness in the 1970's, 1980's, 1990's?'. I do remember once showing one of my poems to a consultant many years ago. She responded to it as if it were an analytical offering. I reckon there is about 40% of who I think I am, including some of the most valuable parts, that psychiatry has either shown no interest in, or has actively brushed aside. I can remember vividly one occasion, about ten years into my career in the mental health system, when I tried to talk to my consultant about what I experienced during psychotic episodes. She didn't want to know. 'Forget about all this stuff' she said. 'It doesn't have any significance. Your brain isn't functioning properly. It's just like when a steam train is running on so fast that its pistons come off.' I believe that was the last time I spoke spontaneously to an expert about my inner world. Looking back now, I can see again what a powerful and menacing set of symbols she dumped on me. The machine that has lost control, that has no proper function. The headlong rush towards something not definable but presumably awful. The flailing pistons. It certainly shut me up good and proper. I seem to remember being thirteen at my final year in prep school, and being handed a little book about riding along in a chariot, pulled by two unruly and powerful horses. I think that was something to do with the dangers of masturbation. That shut me up too. I wonder if there's any connection here?

I believe that telling people, directly or indirectly, that some of their profoundest, most confusing, most distressing, most memorable thoughts, feelings and perceptions are meaningless, and not worth considering, must do more harm than good. I feel personally that part of me was cut adrift and abandoned by such assertions, and by the subsequent lack of interest and imagination my experiences have evoked from most mental health workers. Instead of being offered some possible frameworks within which I could attempt to place a value, and a significance, on my interior realities, I was handed (handed, not offered) one framework which effectively denied that my interior experiences were worthy of valuation. To put it emotionally, and perhaps over-dramatically, I feel that psychiatry has not only insulted my intelligence but also my humanity.

In recent years, there has been much concern about developing mental health services that put the consumer/customer/client/patient/user at the centre, that are individualized, and offer respect and dignity. I think it is unlikely that we will achieve the necessary improvements in care and treatment simply by involving service users on planning committees, or giving users more information about treatments, or independent advocacy services, or even by ensuring fewer people get given the needle against their wishes. However important all these things may be, they will not give people the necessary respect and dignity while the psychiatric approach continues to ignore, or dismiss, significant parts of their lives. How can I make myself whole when the discipline that dominates understanding of the crucial events in my life, refuses to acknowledge large parts of my experience?

I believe psychiatry exhibits a catastrophic lack of sympathetic imagination in its attempts to care for people with diagnoses of psychotic illness. During my own psychotic episodes, I have frequently had powerful and unusual thoughts, feelings and perceptions in relation to God, the Devil, and Jesus Christ. (Given the nature of my upbringing, and the culture and society in which I have lived, this is probably not very surprising.) Although it is more than possible that feelings of connectedness to God, feelings of transcendence if you like, are nothing more than a biochemical spasm in the brain, they have always had a somewhat wider significance for me. Although I am not a member of any religion, I would describe myself as a religious person. Questions about meaning, about good and evil, have not just been symptoms of psychosis in my life.

Moreover, and equally unsurprising I feel, a number of my psychotic episodes (could they be spiritual crises?) have involved external events of a religious nature. Being exorcized by a fellow-patient in an acute ward quiet room, running away from hospital and being found at the foot of the altar in a local church – events of this kind. Yet never, during 20 years of recurrent admissions, did anyone look to draw any conclusions from these events. As I've already indicated, no mental health worker has ever expressed any interest in what I believed in or whether I felt spirituality was important or insignificant. I find such lack of response, such a vacuum in the caring approach to someone in psychosis, quite baffling and disturbing. It implies to me either a total ignorance of what possible may be going on in psychosis, or a major failure of nerve and sympathy. During more recent admissions, I have increasingly sought out priests and chaplains and have found this helpful. But even this has been intermittent interest. I acknowledge that spiritual or religious areas are sensitive, and individual, parts of human life, so that questions of how to make an approach are extremely important and may be difficult to learn. What worries me is that we seem to still to be approaching the stage of asking whether to address this rather than how.

I have used the acute ward of my local asylum four or five times in the last dozen years. It provides me with certain technical assistance to emerge from a crisis: a certain amount of safety, short-term medication, food and rest, a wooden bench among beautiful gardens. These are not to be dismissed. But in other ways, my periods in the asylum are essentially barren. The care I receive makes no attempt to touch certain areas of my life. Questions I now feel are paramount (and have always felt were important) psychiatry does not seek to ask, let alone to answer. I do not look to psychiatry to help me value my life. I don't believe psychiatry is sympathetic to concerns of this nature. Psychiatry, and psychiatrists, have certainly helped me to live my life but, in the process, they have both disregarded and devalued me.

2.15

'THE SERVICE USER'S PERSPECTIVE ON THE CARE PROGRAMME APPROACH'

Questions of identity are important for all of us. They are particularly important for those of us who have a diagnosis of mental illness. This can be illustrated in my position today. A dozen years ago it would hardly have been conceivable that I would be here in this role at this conference. Or that you would be listening to me. What has happened? How much has it changed? Are you really going to listen to me?

There are nowadays a large number of different phrases and terms being used to describe people who would once have been called lunatics and who most people would now call 'the mentally ill'. Some of these terms are the result of people looking for new ways of defining their identity, in particular looking for new ways of giving positive value to dominant aspects of what has been seen as their identity. 'Mental health consumer' or 'mental health service user' are two commonly used phrases. I choose to call myself a 'mental health system survivor', and in my case, this has been a deliberate choice, arrived at over a period of deliberation. Two aspects of this phrase are of major importance to me and, I believe, are worth mentioning at this point. Firstly, I feel strongly that I have had to endure and survive, and am still surviving and enduring, a system of care that has been hostile to me, to my real needs and my wants, to my dignity and my value as a human being and a citizen. I think there are many who share some of that strong feeling. But, more important is the second aspect of the phrase. I feel I am surviving a 'mental health system'. This includes mental health services but is made up of much more than just those. It also includes the entire social and cultural apparatus that has been built up over centuries to capture and cope with the lives and experiences of the mad. Mental health nurses should not ignore this dimension of the lives of people who come to them or are sent to them for help. Mental health services, and using or consuming mental health services, has never been the only concern of those diagnosed as mentally ill. In recent decades, increasingly large areas of the

Presentation by Peter Campbell, founder member of *Survivors Speak Out*, Tuesday 1 August 1995

 DOI: 10.4324/9781003636434-26

life of the 'long-term mentally ill' of whom I am one, have had very little directly to do with mental health services or workers. Anyone who wants to practise the Care Programme Approach (CPA) needs to begin to make a sensitive, and considered, encounter with the real identity, the full identities, of any individual service recipient they come to work with. To what extent are mental health nurses really in sympathy with the lives and experiences, the goals and aspirations, of people with a diagnosis of mental illness?

Not being listened to is a dominant feature of the lives of people with a diagnosis of mental illness. Indeed, it is one defining characteristic of our acquired status. The change from 'mental patient' to 'mental health service consumer' has not substantially altered this. There are a range of reasons why you may discount or devalue what I say now or in future encounters. I am mad, I am not a mental health professional, I am an activist, I am a 'professional user'. This last, convenient because unspecified, description has been a regular way of marginalising the evidence coming from certain service recipients over the last ten years. Leaders of the mental health nursing profession are happy enough to bring it out from time to time. I would challenge anyone who uses this phrase to cast aspersions on my, or other contributors, to the mental health debate to have the courage to spell out their concerns, rather than resort to comfortable posturing. If service providers have concerns about the representativeness of what certain service users are saying – and this seems to be one part of the uneasiness that hides within the negative phrase 'professional user'– they should bring this into the open so that we can all discuss representativeness: but including how representativeness affects the validity of evidence, and how the representativeness of professional users compares with that of professional mental health worker organisations and professional voluntary organisations. At the moment, those with power in mental health services are playing fast and loose with the criteria for involvement. It would be good to know whether we are all playing in the same park, let alone whether the fields there are level.

I doubt whether many service users would oppose the basic package that makes up the Care Programme Approach. Needs-led assessment, a care-planning meeting, a key worker, regular review of the agreed plan are all eminently desirable. They seem to promise recipients a good bit more control over our care and treatment – and this is something that a large number of us are looking for. Indeed (and this is entirely anecdotal evidence) I have yet to meet a mental health service user who did not want more control over their own lives. So, the questions that occur are not over whether the care programme approach is a good idea but whether the CPA mechanism, the CPA process, can deliver the goods. Will the long journey through the Care Programme Approach feel that much better than previous treks through the maze? Will a smoother more involving delivery system alter the stuff on the menu? After CPA, will I get a cup of tea when I arrive after 10:00 PM for a crisis admission? Will I have to answer fewer irrelevant questions? When I get to the day centre at the far end of the journey, will the atmosphere and activities be any less mind-numbing? Method without matter may feel somewhat better but ultimately it is a big con.

Of course, none of us are really able to answer these or other questions about the CPA with much conviction at this stage, standing as we do only a few years into the life of this approach. As an outsider – most user-led organisations do not have the resources to monitor the CPA in a widespread or coherent way – most of what I have to contribute is impressionistic or based on reading official reports and documents. At present, I have two major areas of concern: one regarding the way in which CPA has been implemented so far, and what it is really capable of achieving; and one regarding what CPA might lead to if certain attitudes and beliefs about the care of people with long-term problems come to predominate.

Confusion over language, concepts and terminology seems to have been a feature of the Care Programme Approach so far. It is only slightly unfair to suggest that the most effective method of confusing mental health workers and mental health service users is to devise two approaches to care and treatment, similar but different, call them similar names – Care Programme Approach and Care Management, and try to put them into operation at the same time. I have yet to hear a clear and convincing description of the interaction between the two systems and although the conceptual details may not be of immediate concern to most service recipients, the overall wooliness is not helpful when coordination and information giving is so central to the new systems. Of greater concern, perhaps, is the significant group of recipients who do not know who, or why, their keyworker is.

Commitment is another area where there seems room for doubts. We have been told via a good number of reports over the last year that implementation of the CPA is patchy. Of course, "patchy" is the leitmotif of mental health services at the moment, but even so I don't think that there is much room for contentment about how swiftly CPA is being taken up and put into operation. I recently overheard someone saying that one report suggested that about three quarters of authorities had not got guidelines for the implementation and practise of CPA. If this is true, then I think it does call into question the degree of commitment within the Department of Health and the higher echelons of the mental health services. Anecdotal evidence suggests that numbers of inpatients are still being discharged with sketchy or non-existent plans and that some patients do not have key workers. In the light of the above, I am not at all reassured that short stay patients leaving acute units are really getting a significantly more sensitive service during the period immediately prior to, and following, discharge. The overlooking of the psychological and practical aspects of hospital discharge has always, in my opinion, been a remarkable feature of mental health services. CPA may only do a little to change such a lack of awareness. But if people are leaving in-patient care without plans or key workers, then we really must start considering some much more basic attitudinal flaws.

And what about the quality of care planning, if and when it occurs? There is certainly a danger that we distort and devalue what is going on within the mental health services by focusing too much on the spectacular failures and the intensive reports that result from them – for example, the reports examining the cases of Christopher Clunis, Michael Buchanan and Eileen and Alan Boland. The report on Michael Buchanan is quite scathing on the final Section 117 meeting and follow-up to it in his case. Alongside this I would like to place evidence from a close friend of mine who recently went to a clear planning meeting. Her main concern was that she would be put on the supervision register and as a result would face unwelcome interferences from mental health workers in her life. I will return to this aspect in a moment. But the conduct of the meeting itself was revealing. She said the psychiatrist and the GP spoke to each other about her, and her care, as if she was not even there. It was only when the key worker was involved that my friend's presence was acknowledged, and she became part of the discussion. Then it was back to the psychiatrist and the GP and she ceased to exist again. This is infinitely depressing and suggests that we will have to do much more to change the culture than simply slot in the CPA. Without better training in information-giving, without effective advocacy (both areas, I would suggest, where mental health nurses are under-skilled and complacent) it seems likely that the new approach will feel scarcely more empowering than its predecessors.

I am also worried that the impact of the key worker may not be entirely benign – particularly in the context of inpatient nursing. I have heard reports and myself seen events that suggest key working may encourage nurses who are not key working an individual to disregard their day-to-day needs. In short, we may be encouraging even less general interaction of mental health nurses and in-patients. Some survivors have spoken to me about receiving 'nursing by appointment'. In my view, this is a dreadful development. The main quality of the nursing contribution in such settings is closely linked to the fact that nurses do not just come down to the ward for a few meetings with their clients and then drive off somewhere else. If key working allows more nurses to spend more time in the nursing office and still think they're doing their jobs right, I am totally opposed to it. Perhaps we should be demolishing a few nursing office walls and heralding in a NMHNA – a new mental health nursing approach.

To turn now to some of the add-ons to the basic CPA package – although I recognise the idea of client registers is not exactly new it was quite closely associated with the care programme approach from the outset, it still feels to many of us like an add-on. Supervision registers are not popular with the service users that I know best. Numbers of us live along the boundaries of inclusion within such registers (the fact that in some areas only four people were on the register whereas in other areas everyone in touch with specialist psychiatric services were on it, suggest that the boundaries themselves are currently very moveable indeed). Numbers of us are not satisfied with what mental health services have to offer us and as a result are not looking for more frequent and more insistent visits from people bringing the same shoddy goods. In essence what I would like to see is the CPA being used to give service users a better deal within consistently improving services. The supervision register arrangement of the CPA theme seems quite likely to lead us further down the road towards pressuring people – people who are vulnerable and do not know what is good for them, and obviously mental health services must be good for them – to put up with the unacceptable.

It may irk some people to talk too much about civil and human rights and it is perhaps true that supervision registers represent only a minor erosion of rights.

Nevertheless, it seems quite wrong to me that we should not have the right to appeal to an independent body regarding our inclusion on such lists and completely inappropriate that mental health workers should have leeway over whether they tell people they are on these lists in the first place. In this instance, if you feel distressed because people are watching you more closely, the truth is they are watching you more closely. I was involved as a member of a Community Health Council in discussions about a local register prior to the supervision register proposals. I have to say I was not reassured about health service providers' sensitivity to civil rights and confidentiality issues. It seems ironic to me that at a time when most mental health workers seem so uninterested in improving the reputations of 'the mentally ill' within society, they should seem so casual in letting more and more groups and agencies know who and where we are.

I have campaigned against the proposals to extend compulsory treatment powers into community settings ever since the Hallstrom Case judgement of the mid 1980s. I do not believe that mental health workers need more powers to threaten and compel us. Such powers have many destructive effects, both on those receiving them and those who resort to their use. If mental health workers, including mental health nurses, did their jobs properly and were supported to work in the way they were trained to work, and which they know is the good way, I do not believe there would be a need for aftercare under supervision. You have more than sufficient powers already under the 1983 Mental Health Act. To be blunt, and particularly in the absence of any new resources, it looks like some of us are going to get a lousy deal because of your failings. Now that the government has got round to amendment of the 1983 Act, they have come up with something that nobody appears to want. As a long-term recipient of mental health services, I cannot say that I am particularly surprised at this outcome. On the other hand, it does not lend much lustre to the professions etc. as a whole and has ominous vibrations of what the future might hold.

It is interesting that debates around compulsory treatment in the community, supervision orders, aftercare under supervision should have unearthed the concept of reciprocity. You may have noticed it in one or two Department of Health briefings in the last year or so. I am not totally clear what is being said about reciprocity by the establishment but it seems to be linked to the Care Programme Approach and to the idea of contracts and, in the context of aftercare under supervision (which to my surprise some are seeing as just a logical extension of the CPA), to an idea that if you take something away from someone like their liberty, you should give them something in return (like a piece of paper with a detailed care plan on it). While in general terms this seems interesting and potentially helpful even, I believe it needs close monitoring. Reciprocity appears to be the very thing that aftercare under supervision is not offering its recipients. Firstly, it will not be a contract freely entered into. Second, while it is quite clear what may happen if the supervisee stops taking their medication, or even does not turn up at the day centre, it is not clear what happens if service providers renege on their part of the bargain. It will take a bit more than rhetorical nods to reciprocity to convince recipients that this type of give and take is benevolent.

Many survivors are strongly in favour of mutuality. Mental health nurses should reflect on the huge growth of self-help initiatives in the field over the last 20 years. They should accept as fundamental that the so-called mentally ill have a lot to give. To nurses, to society, to each other. Professional care givers disempower us too often because they are too arrogant, too inflexible, too afraid, to allow such exchanges to take place. Each time I hear, and read about, Treatment Compliance – and I read about it very frequently in the *Nursing Times* these days – I wince. You have an enormous investment in keeping us inferior and passive. In keeping us wrong.

In the conference notes, I put the question that 'You cannot fix the water supply by fiddling with the tap'? Of course, the tap does control the supply – so you can fix it that way. And this is in a large part what the Care Programme Approach is setting out to do. Questions about how much water is getting through, and who is the flow being principally directed at, are not unimportant. But for me, the real concern should be over the quality of the water, and whether we shouldn't be doing more to fix that. I believe we should be asking those with the thirst about whether they want water or cola syrup or even chloral hydrate syrup coming out of the tap. Although I believe a nice warm shower is better than a short burst below the waistline, I think that is a less important concern.

The Care Programme Approach is essentially a mechanism. A mechanism that will be controlled by the attitudes and assumptions of those with power over it. While I hope mental health nurses will learn the best skills to operate CPA most sensitively and effectively, I feel the important struggle lies elsewhere – to discover the true humanity of the mad without destroying all their difference, to fight alongside service users for their reputation in society, to recapture through mutual enquiry the real skills of the mental health nurse.

2.16

'THROUGH THE REVOLVING DOOR' (1999)

Introduction

I have had 20 admissions into acute psychiatric wards since 1967. Two-thirds were carried through under sections of the Mental Health Acts 1959 or 1983. In many respects, this is a record in which I myself, and those charged with my care and treatment, can take little pride. At one level, it cannot help but seem like (and actually be) a record of failure. But, on the other hand, at least I am still here. At least the caring team has been able to contain me during crisis and return me quite rapidly to life in the community. And to do that consistently, for more than 30 years. At one level, that seems like (and actually is) quite a success. In the 1970s, I often felt that my crises would destroy me. At some point thereafter, I lost that fear – a significant liberation for which the NHS acute psychiatric ward is in no small way responsible. As a psychiatric dressing station, the acute ward has rendered me valuable service over the years. It is my contention that it could, and should, be something more.

Going in

Winning greater control over care and treatment has been one important element in action by the service user/survivor movement since the 1980s. And crisis services have regularly been a focus for concern. Service users are often at their most powerless during crises, both as a result of the intensity of their own distress and because mental health workers can take that distress as a reason to ignore, or devalue, their wishes. While complete avoidance of crisis may be a legitimate, and realisable, goal for many people with a mental illness diagnosis, for others, myself included, the quality of our journey through crisis and, often, into the acute ward becomes a prime concern.

I believe it is frequently unclear what priority crisis services place on maximising an individual's control during periods of distress. While the widespread use of terminology like 'crisis' would seem to suggest a more positive framework within which to approach people's distress, it does not necessarily guarantee that crisis

 DOI: 10.4324/9781003636434-27

services are working in novel ways, let alone looking at crisis as a time of exploration and learning relevant to the continuing development of the individual. The crisis service I have been using for the last fifteen years has always had a medical orientation. Although it has become a means by which I have won control of my crises, that has been more by effort than design.

Certainly, for my first fifteen years of using psychiatric acute wards, gaining control of my crises was a low priority. This was partly because I was living in inner London, a long distance from the psychiatric hospital I used, and because I moved home regularly. These factors certainly made pre-crisis planning more difficult. But it was also a result of the framework within which my crises appeared to be viewed by the experts. They were essentially 'relapses'– the re-emergence of an underlying and ever-present psychotic illness, against which the only sure defence was regular medication. The standard comment during the first two weeks of every admission was always 'So, you stopped taking your tablets did you?' I was sold the idea that I was the victim of a cyclical illness that would almost inevitably re-occur. Short of taking medication as prescribed, I was given little or no guidance on how to avoid future crises. Most of what I did learn was in spite of, rather than because of, mental health services. At the same time, I experienced 'drugging out' or 'zapping' on a number of occasions – where you are drugged into unconsciousness within an hour or so of arrival on the acute ward. I remember being 'drugged out' once in the middle of the admission procedure, waking up in a following shift, and having to start the procedure all over again. It is possible that 'drugging out' is a legitimate intervention and I can remember times when its use on me was justifiable. But it often appeared to be used indiscriminately. I remember being 'drugged out' after having been brought in by the local police and strongly resisting admission. Then, returning by myself to the same hospital less than twelve months later, and negotiating my own admission, only to be drugged out in exactly the same way. I would hesitate to call such treatment anti-therapeutic but it certainly penalised personal development. Above all, it reminded me just who was really in control of my distress and just how powerful they were.

The service user/survivor movement in the United Kingdom has been campaigning for almost 20 years for non-medical crisis services. Originally, that seems to have meant crisis services along the lines of Soteria House and Diabasis in the United States (Mosher and Burti, 1994) where medication was not used. Subsequently, and with the growth of the movement, non-medical seems to have shifted to mean services where the medical model does not dominate, and where medication is used sparingly and not as a first resort. It certainly implies no compulsory medication. But the use, or non-use, of medication which was a defining issue in the early 1980s, seems to have become less central, provided other components, what might be called an 'holistic' approach to crisis, are included in services. The belief that large numbers of people can journey through crisis without medication, although still an important element in many survivor activists' approach to distress, has not convinced the mainstream service providers.

My own attitude to the use of medication during crisis is pragmatic. Although I want always to use the least medication possible, the fact that I know short-term doses of neuroleptics will bring me out of a crisis very rapidly is both extremely reassuring in ordinary times and of practical benefit during distress. Having said that, I can see the advantage in terms of feelings of self-esteem, autonomy and integrity attached to journeying successfully through the crisis without medication. While at this stage in my life, I do not have a particular desire to go through a crisis without medication, I support the creation of suitable resources for people who do. For me, the important issue in relation to the use of medication in crisis is not use, or non-use, but appropriate and sensitive use. I would particularly like to see restraints on the power of mental health workers to administer heavy doses of psychiatric drugs. 'Drugging out' is not the only example of insensitive prescribing. Many acute ward users can remember the humiliation of drug-induced semi-consciousness that can be a feature of their first few days on the ward. Whether such practices serve the interests of the ward staff, or the persons in crisis, is hard to tell. Service users consistently report that information about medication is inadequate (Campbell et al., 1998) and it is currently almost impossible for an in-patient to know if they are receiving the optimal dosages. I have always found medication to be the most sensitive area when trying to collaborate with mental health workers around my own crisis care. Questioning the psychiatrist's expertise in this area is extremely difficult. It took me 20 years to win agreement that I should be given one neuroleptic in crisis as opposed to another (essentially similar). The next time I was admitted I was still given the drug they had promised not to give me. It is possible to place too much emphasis on medication and other physical treatments and procedures (like solitary confinement) because they exemplify, in the starkest way, the individual's loss of control on their journey through the revolving door. But you can be demolished as well by the caring team's mind-set as by an Acuphase injection. If the much-vaunted partnership of service user and mental health worker is to be an actual rather than a rhetorical one, it is always likely to be unequal. Medication is only one of a number of areas where it may be particularly unbalanced.

Over the last fifteen years, the service user/survivor movement has promoted advocacy as a principal weapon in moderating imbalances of power and times of crises have naturally been seen as occasions when independent advocacy may be particularly necessary. The first Crisis Card, launched by the International Self Advocacy Alliance in 1989, at a time when there were relatively few mental health advocacy services, was a practical way for people to nominate an advocate and have that recognised. It was also a device to highlight the inadequacy of crisis services that made advocacy so necessary. For the producers of the original Crisis Card, as for the majority of their successors, the need for advocacy has always been due more to the failings of the service than the distress of the service user.

Unfortunately, it is very difficult to assess the usefulness of crisis cards. Although one or two local areas have kept records, there has been no systematic study of how they have been used, whether they have been used and how helpful they have been. While there are a few places where the use of crisis cards has been agreed by the relevant agencies (police, social services, health services), in other areas it has been left to individual service users to negotiate their own agreement with the mental health workers connected with their care. My own crisis card is entered into the computer of the acute ward I use. Although that system has proved notoriously unreliable in the past, it is significant and useful to me that the services I know have an advocate and have recognised her legitimacy. On the other hand, I have never used the card to call my advocate to help and it is still unclear how frequently crisis cards are being used in this way.

It would certainly be interesting to know more about how advocates are used during crisis. How many times are advocates supporting a partner before they are admitted into a crisis house or acute ward and how often are they only coming into contact with potential partners once they have been admitted? Given that the Mental Health Act Code of Practice Continues to give rather lukewarm advice to Approved Social Workers about the involvement of advocates in assessment procedures, can we assume that most advocates become involved with 'detained patients' after rather than during the event? Is the journey through crisis prior to arrival in services essentially an advocacy-free zone? Again, it is very difficult to assess the nature and usefulness of crisis advocacy because, although the evidence is presumably there, it hasn't been published in any consolidated way. There is a certain irony in the fact that as the service user survivor movement and others line up to press for the inclusion of the right to advocacy in a new Mental Health Act, we are to some extent promoting a pig in a poke.

Having someone who can help you speak out for what you want during crisis is a valuable advantage (I will never forget how bringing my advocate into the multidisciplinary ward round for the first time completely transformed the dynamics of the meeting). Finding some way of influencing in advance the care and treatment you will receive is even better. Extending the care programme so that it includes details of what will happen if you are in crisis, and in particular what treatment you will be given on the acute ward, is one possibility. Having a separate crisis plan agreed with the acute ward is another. Whether these give the individual any greater control at the time of admission rather than retrospectively, is a debatable question. For a number of service users, the way forward is through advance directives that carry legal weight. At present, a person with a mental illness diagnosis and decision-making capacity can be detained and treated against their will. They can make legally binding advance directives about treatment for their physical health but not their mental health. In these circumstances, the extent to which anyone in a mental health crisis can be in control of their treatment must be significantly circumscribed. The only way to alter the situation is to change our status under statute law.

The non-compliance of mental health workers with agreed treatment programmes is likely to be an issue during and after the development of new mental health legislation. Already there have been calls from a number of professionals for the introduction of advance directives into legislation (Szmukler, 1999) and a suggestion that the provisions of any Care Programme should be mandatory. It is clear many in the service use/survivor movement see advantages in such a 'contractual' approach to service use. Individuals would certainly have more influence over what was going to happen to them and that could be particularly valuable at times of crisis. They would also have greater opportunities for redress. But the impact it would have on the quality of care is unclear – it could be argued that contractual care will be minimum standards/defensive care. Moreover, this approach might do little or nothing to alter the overall shape of services. I do not see any individual crisis plan of mine creating services ex nihilo. Like advocacy and advance directives, it is essentially a protection in the light of a service that does not meet my needs.

Being in

While it may be unfair to talk about the failure of the psychiatric acute ward, there is no doubt that perceptions of its unsuitability as a destination for people in distress have been a central element in action by service user/survivors over the last 20 years and that these perceptions have recently become more widespread. The Sainsbury Centre for Mental Health's *Acute Problems*, a survey of the quality of care in acute psychiatric wards (The Sainsbury Centre for Mental Health, 1998) which includes as one of its core conclusions that 'Hospital care is a nontherapeutic intervention', is anticipated in many respects by *Treated Well? A Code of Practice for Psychiatric Hospitals* (Good Practices in Mental Health/Camden Consortium, 1988), one of the first publications from a local service user/survivor group produced ten years earlier. If the psychiatric acute ward is in crisis, it has been a long crisis.

Reading the above reports is a reminder of the extent to which the physical surroundings and basic amenities on acute wards have been, and continue to be, inadequate. Of 112 patients interviewed at time of discharge in the Sainsbury centre study, 55% had no separate bedrooms; 71% no secure locker for belongings; 47% had no quiet place in which to meet visitors; 20% felt washing facilities were not private; 32% did not feel safe on the wards. Leaving aside the nature of their distress, it is not difficult to see why service users find acute wards unpleasant places to be.

The acute ward based in a remote and slowly declining asylum, or in the inner-city District General Hospital unit, cramped and confined, are two images of the acute ward in the 1980s and 1990s. There must be qualified optimism that we can avoid their recreation in the next decades. Certainly, after years of being told that 'this place isn't a hotel, you know', it is gratifying to discover that a Royal College of Psychiatrists working party (Royal College of Psychiatrists, 1998) has argued that accommodation on newly built acute units should 'bear comparison with a comfortable modern hotel'. Official guidance also recommends single bedrooms with en suite toilet facilities for all patients. The question seems to be whether and when we will be building new acute wards.

Acute Problems cites a number of reasons for its conclusion that hospital care is a non-therapeutic intervention. One factor may be the number and quality of interactions between professionals and acute ward users. Outside of nurses and psychiatrists, these averaged at less than one per patient per 38-day average stay. Furthermore, the report when taken alongside the Mental Health Act Commission and Sainsbury Centre National Visit (*Mental Health Act Commission*, 1997) lends support to the longstanding anecdotal evidence that psychiatric nurses' interaction with acute ward users has changed over the last fifteen years. Nurses do appear to spend less time talking to acute ward users, partly because there are fewer nurses, because a greater proportion are forced or choose to spend time in the nursing office, because other duties divert them from being in the day areas.

Observation is an important element in this change. It appears to have become more common, partly in response to higher levels of distress among people admitted onto acute wards, partly in response to greater sensitivity to risk among service providers. As a result, there is a tendency for the direction of nursing care to be diverted. As Adams and Kennedy (*Psychiatric Bulletin* Jan 1988) say:

> 'So it is not just that the policy of level one observation is transforming the culture of psychiatric wards from therapeutic to custodial, which may in itself raise risks, it is also that the flexibility of nursing staff to monitor and respond to the needs of all patients under their care is so reduced as to give a lot to the few and virtually nothing to the majority.'
>
> (p.57)

It has long been clear that acute ward users find talking to people helpful, although they have often found other users more helpful than psychiatric nurses. Now that there is evidence that nurses are increasingly dropping out of the equation, a number of suggestions have been put forward. One that has already been tried in many places is 'nursing by appointment', where each person has the right to a certain amount of time with a key nurse. While this might heighten the value each party places on the interaction, it does not necessarily produce the desired communication and may actually reduce the amount of interaction with other nurses in the ward. A further suggestion in the *National Visit* (1997) was that nurses needed specialised skills to deal with people diagnosed with psychotic illnesses and should have more training in cognitive behavioural and similar interventions.

Although there may be a case for turning psychiatric nurses into therapists, it is also worth encouraging them to communicate more often, and more generally, with acute ward users. Perhaps more research should be done on what sort of talking and listening acute ward users find helpful, and why they find talking with fellow users so important. It is unlikely to be provided by sessional nursing. In 1972, I spent four months in an acute ward where the nurses came out of the office, where we had a ward meeting every weekday morning that discussed people's lives, not withdrawals from the patients' bank, and where there was a real feeling of community. It seemed like a place where something useful was going on. For the last fifteen years, the acute ward has seemed to me to be a place where nothing was really happening. Whether we rescue the psychiatric acute ward by bringing mental health workers and acute ward users into a more effective community or by fragmenting them into individual therapeutic relationships is one possible issue for the future.

'It's not the real you'

Unsurprisingly, there is evidence that mental health workers and acute ward users do not always look at things in the same way. One survey (Sharma et al., 1992) found significant differences between nursing staff and patients over what was most helpful. For example, while nurses felt 'staff-intensive' measures were most beneficial for patients, patients found them no more useful than 'non-staff-intensive' measures. Patients rated drug treatment and ward rounds in their bottom four of helpful items Nursing staff placed them in their top four. A later review (Sainsbury Centre for Mental Health, 1998) shows that acute ward users at admission place greater emphasis on social needs and, among other differences, found that only 12% agreed with staff about having psychotic problems. It is possible that findings of this kind are an indication of differences on other levels.

The phrase 'It's not the real you....' has been a common accompaniment of my time in acute wards over the last 30 years. Spoken sometimes as a comfort, as a control, as a dismissal, this phrase symbolises for me the way mental health workers seek to separate themselves and me from aspects of my distress. Anything psychotic of course cannot be played with (collusion). But whole areas of experience seem immaterial on the acute ward. What do you believe in? And how does it feel to live with a mental illness diagnosis? These are questions I have never heard asked. The possibility that people may be wanting to integrate problematic aspects of themselves, rather than cutting them off, subordinating or subduing them, is not entertained.

Edward Podvoll (1990, p.65) has described an 'asylum mentality' which he feels makes recovery from psychosis more difficult. Its characteristics include what has been called the 'silence that humiliates', a studied interpersonal rift between doctor and patient designed to make the patient reflect on madness. Without endorsing Podvoll's view, it does seem that a huge silence has fallen over the acute ward, that certain areas of experience are not open to exploration, and acute ward users who want to discover the meaning and significance of their distress will not be encouraged.

Ultimately, I have not found the separation of feeling and perception (unreal meaningless) and behaviour (significant, preventable) during my 'psychotic episodes' to be helpful. While the acute ward can contain and adjust the latter efficiently, each new admission is an essentially barren experience. To an extent, the implication that the content of psychosis and the whole crisis itself is somehow at one remove from the real is actually destructive. I am certainly not attracted to madness. Although society believes madness can be attractive, I have personally never met an acute ward user who expressed the desire to 'get mad again'. Instead, I have found many, myself included, who believe the capacity for madness is worth integrating into rather than alienating from their lives. For us, the declaration 'It's not the real you...' is first and foremost an act of therapeutic aggression.

There are signs that some of the new crisis services are attempting to move away from the divisive approach to distress that has characterised many medically-dominated services. An 'holistic' approach to distress and 'letting the individual define their crisis' sound like a stronger invitation to exploration and self-understanding. If this is indeed the case, one important question that arises (certainly from the viewpoint of someone like myself) is: can these new methods be transferred to the acute ward?

At present, there appears to be a feeling that the numbers of people (staff and acute ward users) involved in most acute wards, and the hierarchies associated with size, would make much of the innovative work in alternative crisis facilities impossible (Mosher, 1999). If that is true, the important question becomes: how do you prevent the creation of a two-tier crisis service – with innovative care in crisis houses for those with the right type of distress and second-class care in acute wards for those (e.g., people on sections) whose distress does not fit?

Ultimately, I believe that my distress/madness/psychosis is the real me. I feel crisis is a suitable time to consider that inter-relatedness. The acute wards I have used, have, by and large, refuted both those propositions and have concentrated on getting me back together and out into the community again. A role, I readily acknowledge, it does very efficiently. But with no soul. It seems to me that size should not prevent acute ward care from touching the spirits of service users more tenaciously. We would not be breaking any professional codes if we acknowledged that something important was going on in crisis that was not to do with illness. In the acute wards of the next decade, it would be good to see psychosis come out of the shrouds – something we could discuss without succumbing....

References

Adams, R., Kennedy, P. (1998) Letter in *Psychiatric Bulletin* 22 (57).

Campbell, P., Cobb, A., Darton, K. (1998) 'Psychiatric Drugs: Users' Experiences and Current Policy and Practice', MIND.

Good Practices in Mental Health/Camden Consortium (1988) *Treated Well: A Code of Good Practise for Psychiatric Hospitals*. GPMH.

Mental Health Act Commission and Sainsbury Centre for Mental Health (1997) *The National Visit*. Sainsbury Centre.

Mosher, L., Burti, M. (1994) *Community Mental Health: A Practical Guide*. Norton.

Mosher, L. (1999) Presentation at *Mental Health Foundation*, 8 January 1999.

Podvoll, E. (1990) *The Seduction of Madness*. Century.

Royal College of Psychiatrists (1998) *Not Just Bricks and Mortar*. Royal College of Psychiatrists.

Sharma T., Carson J., Berry, C. (1992) 'Patient Voices', *Health Service Journal* 16 (1992) pp. 20–21.

Sainsbury Centre for Mental Health (1998) 'Acute Problems: A Survey of the Quality of Care in Acute Psychiatric Wards', Sainsbury Centre.

Szmukler, G. (1999) Cited in *Community Care*, 25–31 March 1999.

2.17

'BACK TO CAMBRIDGE'
[*Testimony* 2000]

'I arrived back at Cambridge, but I was done really. I was finished. Because I'd had ECT, I was on large doses, by that time, of Chlorpromazine, and in the final year I had to study medieval Latin for one of my papers. It was quite a long time since I'd looked at Latin, and medieval Latin's not the same as classical Latin. And, basically, I couldn't...I realized half-way through the following term, about February time, that there was no way I could do it. I was sitting in the university library staring, and I couldn't concentrate. I was gone. And I was drugged up to the eyeballs as well. So, basically, I hauled up the surrender flag and I got admitted into Fulbourn Hospital, which is the big psychiatric hospital outside Cambridge, and I spent the rest of that year in Fulbourn and ended up getting a special class of degree, what they call an aegrotat degree, so I got an honours degree, but I didn't sit the final exams.

Cambridge was for me a very difficult period in my life. One of the things is that, if you're becoming a mental patient or becoming a loony, if you like, to use that phrase, it isolates you from other people, and when I think of my experience of having these episodes, and ending up in psychiatric hospital, they were bound to isolate me from other people. Not only do you fall through your year so you end up in another year, but you actually feel significantly different from other people, who have gone straight from successful life in a public school or grammar school to a successful life at a top university. I'd kind of fallen out of that model, and that's partly what becoming a mental patient is about – you lose your expectations of yourself, of what you're capable of, of what's possible for you, and you also lose contact with the expectations of your peers.

DOI: 10.4324/9781003636434-28

2.18

'THE EXPERIENCE OF SECLUSION'. [*Testimony* 2000]

'When I was first admitted to West Park Mental Hospital, in Epsom I was in quite severe distress, so I got admitted to the admission ward and then, after about a week, I was transferred to a locked ward and ended up in solitary confinement. In retrospect, they said that they couldn't cope with me on the open ward because, apparently, I kept throwing myself out of my bed. On one or two occasions, they had just settled me on my bed, and gone away, and they heard this tremendous thump, and they'd turn around and go back into the ward and I'm kind of lying on the floor. So, basically, I was obviously quite agitated, and so I think they decided that I'd have to go to a locked ward. I was put in seclusion, solitary confinement, and then I went on hunger strike. I think that was certainly partly, maybe even largely, because I'd been put in seclusion, and it may also have been because of other things that were going on in my personal drama. Anyway, I went on hunger strike, and they had to delegate a nurse to try and persuade me to eat, and she used to come in every so often into the seclusion room, trying to persuade me to drink and eat. I was in there for a couple of days or so, I suppose, in seclusion.

I tried to batter my way out of the seclusion room, which isn't a very clever idea. I mean, I injured my shoulder, not permanently, but it certainly wasn't, you know, a nice experience being locked up in this kind of bare room with a mattress on the floor, being in your underclothes, basically, and a cardboard piss pot, and people coming every so often to see if you're okay, and two people standing by the door, shoulder to shoulder, kind of talking to you. If you're not already feeling pretty paranoid, that kind of experience is enough to make you feel that way anyway.

I also had the extraordinary incident of being interviewed for benefit while I was in seclusion, because I'd written a letter, as soon as I got admitted, asking about benefit. And the benefit woman from the Epsom office came up, and kind of interviewed me, while I was sitting on the seclusion room floor in my underpants. It's one of those surreal things, and I've still got the letter at home that she sent to me afterwards saying, 'You may remember that I visited you on such and such and you appeared to be saying such and such…'. It was just really, really weird but at least she was trying to attend to some of my needs, which is probably more than a lot of the nursing staff were doing really. In the end, I then spent a period of time

DOI: 10.4324/9781003636434-29

on the locked ward, with the hard cases, if you like, and with the cutlery being counted, you know, before and after each meal, and all that kind of number, and then eventually went back to Emerson ward, the admission ward I'd come from. I then went into a period of being given large quantities of medication and then, when that didn't seem to be working well enough, I was given ECT. After about two or three months, I was OK again, and then this idea about the therapeutic community was put forward.

I think there may not have been much alternative to putting me into seclusion. I think it would have been very difficult for them to supervise me on an open ward. My argument over that particular episode of seclusion, and ones that I've experienced since then, is what do mental health workers do to support people who are in seclusion, and after they've come out of seclusion? Certainly, nobody's ever come up to me and said, 'How do you feel about all this? Do you want to talk if through? How does it make you feel about yourself as a person that this has been done to you? Are you angry about it?' There are a lot of implications about being put in seclusion. You've lost control. You've lost control to such an extent that human beings can't contain you, they've got to throw you into a room with no furniture, and lock you away, until you get a grip on yourself.

All these sorts of messages are important ones that people think about, well I certainly think about. And it seems to me that nurses, and other mental health workers, should be spending time giving people a chance to talk about these things, and come to terms with the experience of being secluded. So, it's not a question about whether it's right or wrong, it's a question about whether or not the caring professions are actually doing enough to counteract what can be an extremely damaging experience. I mean, I've never got over being put in solitary confinement. It's not something I will ever forget, and it's not something that I find it easy to come to terms with even after 30 years being in the system, and possibly I never will. But possibly, if people had talked to me a bit more about it at the time, it might have been easier to actually integrate into my experience. So that was solitary confinement.'

'You prefer to call it solitary confinement rather than seclusion?
'Yeah, because that's what it is. I mean seclusion make it sound like, you know, sitting by the banks of a river with a packet of sandwiches and a good book, which it's not. I mean, it is solitary confinement. I mean, it's about locking people up on their own.

I think there's also another side to solitary confinement. You can look at solitary confinement symbolically, as some kind of rock bottom, if you like, in the psychotic experience. You could argue that maybe it's necessary sometimes for people, and sometimes for me, to go into distress so deeply that in the end you end up in seclusion, in solitary confinement, on your own in a bare room, and that's the kind of rock bottom of your psychotic journey, and then you come out from that. I think there is an element in that you could argue is useful, and I think to some extent that may have been useful to me. You know, maybe there is value in that, in terms of what's going on in people's inner dramas, but even so, it's a powerful experience that people need to be supported through.

I mean it's an important event. I was trained to work with pre-school children, so being violent, and out of control, as a man, and being dealt with in violent restraint kind of ways, is extremely important. I mean the fact that I lose control, it means a lot to me, particularly when it used to happen when I was working, earning my living, working with pre-school children. It's got enormous significance. And for nobody to actually have the imagination to actually talk about it, so you carry this thing round with you. Nobody mentions it, partly because people are guilty about it. It's because mental health workers know that it's wrong and it's a failure. It happens because other things have failed, that's why people end up in seclusion, in solitary confinement. Because it's a failure, mental health workers don't want to look at it. They don't feel happy about what they've had to do, and it's difficult to go to somebody and say 'look, you know, this is what we did to you, and we know it was….let's talk about it'. Instead, what I used to get, on a couple of occasions when I was let out of seclusion, they said, 'Well, we did it for your own good…', which seems to me far too pat an answer. It's getting nurses off the hook, it puts responsibility on you, and leaves all the important questions unanswered.

2.19

'BEING ON SECTION'.
[*Testimony* 2000]

I think the difficulty for me, that has shaped my experience of mental health service, is that I go very rapidly from being OK to not being OK and that quite often means that I get sectioned. I get admitted under compulsion. So that, certainly from the mid-1970s onwards, most of my admissions have been under sections of the Mental Health Act. And that clearly is a problem. Sometimes it's a question of losing a degree of control and going out into the street or the road and doing something that draws attention. You know, stopping the traffic, and where I live in Cricklewood, actually going out in the rush hour and standing in the road by the traffic lights, and just actually preventing the traffic from going. Picking fights on the street, getting very agitated and calling out in the streets., and making loud speeches or exclamations outside cafes in Cricklewood or Kilburn, all that kind of thing. So that may mean that the police are called, and I get admitted under Section 136. Alternatively, if that doesn't happen, I may be sectioned by the crisis team and go in without the police. If the police are involved, I have to go to the police station and then one of the ordeals is that you end up in a police station cell. You're basically getting solitary confinement again when you're kind of in the pit of your distress. You're waiting for the team to come out to assess you. To me that is totally unacceptable, that we should be doing that to people. I don't see that police stations are suitable to detain people in great distress. It should be outlawed. It certainly traumatised me on a couple of occasions. I mean, on one occasion I was put in a police cell and I was pretty out of it, and feeling very negative about myself, and they had left – there was a toilet, you know, it was an open toilet in the cell, you know– somebody had left bleach in the toilet. And I actually washed the whole cell, and myself, in bleach because of the way I was feeling. I was very lucky actually, because when they actually did get me into hospital, they realised. Somebody said, 'What's all this stuff all over him?' And I had got my eyes coated with bleach. They managed to get it all off, and I had to go to see the eye specialist the following day from the acute ward. It was OK. I mean, that's a dramatic example. But I think it's just not appropriate, to have to use seclusion in hospitals. It's certainly not appropriate to have police cells being used as a place of safety, when you can build other facilities, even in a police station.

 DOI: 10.4324/9781003636434-30

And, of course, the problem is, once you're in hospital on a section your liberties are restricted. I suppose there are two things that affect me in that respect. One is your freedom of movement. On a section, it's going to take you longer before you actually get allowed off the ward to go for a walk and then quite often what you have to do is to go through this endless reporting routine. You want to go up to the cafe at Napsbury, so you've got to go into the nursing office, talk to the nurse in charge and say 'please nurse, I want to go off the ward'. Where are you going? I'm going to the cafe. How long are you going to be? I'm going to be 20 minutes. Go, come back, come into the ward again. You say, 'I'm back'. That goes on day after day, you know, while you're on section.

The other thing is that you're not, you can never win an argument when you're on a section, you know. If there's a discussion of any kind about your care and treatment, or about your behaviour, they can say 'well this is the way it is you're on the section', so you just feel even more powerless than you normally would. It does, actually, just aggravate your feeling of powerlessness, and it aggravates the kind of negative side of some of the routines. I remember at Elgar ward at West Park, when they put me on a section, and it was one of the first times that I'd ever been on a section, and what I did every day for a week was, abscond I suppose is the word, at lunchtime because there're two hours between lunch and OT. OT started at 2:00 and lunch finished at 12:15. So what I would do is, I would have my lunch and then I would go, and I would see how far I could walk away from Epsom District Hospital psychiatric unit and get back by 2:00 and, as I say, I did that every day for a week. Well, pretty pointless but I mean it was just a protest. I mean it's the first time I have probably told anybody about it, but it's the way I felt for myself of protesting, the fact that I was on a section, and why I was on a section, but I was quite responsible enough to be allowed out, and I would go and come back, you never tell anybody, so those are some of the kind of to me irritations of being on a section, it's just that you feel you're not in control, you're being treated like a little kid when it's not necessary.

2.20

'AT THE RICHMOND FELLOWSHIP'.
[*Testimony* 2000]

'After waiting until, I think, the late summer of 1973, I then went to a therapeutic community, the Richmond Fellowship in West London, and was there for a year, and that was very different. I think that I was on the verge of becoming a community mental patient by that point, because I hadn't got a profession, I hadn't got a career, I'd spent a lot of time in the previous two or three years in psychiatric hospitals, including a year at West Park, and if somebody had said to me 'What's your profession?', I might well have said, 'Community Mental Patient'. I was beginning to feel, perhaps this is real life, living in an asylum, so that going to the therapeutic community was quite important in as much as they wouldn't take on that stuff. I kind of started off talking to my counsellor within the community sort of saying, 'Oh, I'm a manic depressive, I'm a long term mental patient', you know all that kind of stuff, and she sort of said, 'Oh I'm not interested in all that, we believe that you can take control of your life and we don't want to know about all these labels that are getting you off the hook of doing that'. So, I think that was important psychologically. The year in the therapeutic community didn't in any way prevent me from going in and out of psychiatric hospitals and units, but it did make me feel, well actually I can sort my life, or I can make a good try at it, rather than give in and go on to the community mental patient circuit'.

'What was the set up at the Richmond Fellowship?'

'Right, it was a hostel for about fifteen to twenty people. It was basically for anybody from seventeen to sixty-five, with any type of problem, any type of diagnosis. It was the training house for the Richmond Fellowship at that time, so it was one of their flagship communities, if you like, and it was run as a community. We had a community meeting of the whole house once a week, we had small groups or therapeutic groups, with two staff members, and then each of us had a staff member as an individual counsellor. Then there were various kinds of work groups, to do various aspects of the domestic chores, the cooking, the cleaning, that kind of thing. The idea was that we were running the community, which of course wasn't true. I mean, there was a lot of mystification that went on, that we had the power, the

DOI: 10.4324/9781003636434-31

residents had the power, where we didn't have the power. When it came to certain things, there were certain rules that were laid down by the staff that we couldn't change. For example, if somebody was involved in a violent incident and was the instigator of the violence, they had to leave the house, even if all the other residents felt there were mitigating circumstances. That was basically a rule, there were a number of rules, in actual fact. So, it was partly, being kind of cynical about it, a lot of kind of hiding of the power relationship. In an asylum, it's fairly clear who's got the power and who hasn't got the power, and it's fairly open. In a therapeutic community, I think there's a lot of mystification, a lot of sometimes psychotherapeutic gobbledegook that can be used to make sure that the staff have the power and the residents don't, or only have the feeling that they're in power.

But having said that, it was a very good experience for me, a very useful experience, a very intense experience. I mean, a lot happened. People throwing themselves out of windows and committing suicide. There were two or three suicides while I was there, and people getting into great distress and calling emergency meetings in the middle of the night, and everybody going down. It was very involving, and while I was there it was my world and there was very little that went on outside. A criticism could be that it was supposed to be a half-way house as well, that you were going from there to live in your own place, and in some ways it was such an intense experience that a lot of people weren't really able to prepare themselves for actually leaving. But I learnt a lot, I think, from actually being there, and I made two or three really good friends, in fact my oldest friend from London days is someone I met at that therapeutic community, and a couple of staff members as well I'm still in contact with. So, yeah, it was positive!'

'It sounds very different from all the hospital experiences?'

'Yes, I mean because you were living, there was much more closeness between the staff and the residents, there wasn't this kind of hierarchy that you have in a psychiatric hospital, a distance between the mental health workers and the patients. That was much less so in the therapeutic community'.

'Do you think that sort of place could have been more helpful earlier in your career?'

'Possibly. I think, if you go right back to the beginning, I think if I had not gone back to Scotland, and stayed outside the psychiatric system in some way, that might have made a crucial difference. I think that, at that my point, my distress wasn't very deep, and I think if I'd had some other kind of intervention along the talking, interacting side, that might well have put me on a completely different path. Whereas I think the fact that I kind of got referred into the psychiatric acute ward approach to my problems, although very understandable why it should happen, I think in a way that was probably going in at the deep end, and it then kind of tipped my whole expectation of how this problem should be dealt with along that particular line. I think there's a strong argument for saying that people, myself included, would benefit from talking first before medicating. I think once you start medicating people then you've got to make up a lot of lost ground. It's better to talk first, and medicate afterwards, rather than the other way round'.

2.21

'ALTERNATIVE THERAPIES'
[*Testimony* 2000]

When I was at the Richmond Fellowship I started to get involved in, I suppose you'd call humanistic therapies, encounter groups, bio-energetics groups, those sorts of things, which were being promoted in London at the time. There was a kind of explosion of those kinds of activities. Well, it was a very mixed experience for me because it was totally unregulated. You could simply go along and say, "I want to enroll for this particular encounter group", and basically you would be asked a few simple questions about your background, and sometimes about whether you were taking psychiatric medications and if so what. But I'd never heard of anybody actually being turned down because they were taking a psychiatric medication. I think the difficulty was that the groups could be made up of a very wide range of people, some of whom were just ordinary young people wanting to meet other young people, and do something interesting and interactive with them, and then there were some people who might have particular problems they worked on. And then there was probably a minority, like myself, who actually already had long-term major problems, and some of us had experience of being on the receiving end of psychiatry, and it could leave you wide open. I mean, I got a lot of positive things from it, but I also started to come across real difficulties. Once, for example, I was the one who was doing the work in the group, and it was kind of an assertion exercise where the other members of the group make a line, and they link arms across the room, and you are encouraged to force your way through this line to the other side. And I gave up, and basically sat down on the floor in a corner. And then the group pressure came, you know, "why did you do that? You're not assertive enough!" There was a stereotype already of me in the group as a not particularly assertive person. And I said, Well, have you ever been in seclusion, and have you ever tried to battle your way out of a seclusion door? And I started to think after that, well hang on a second, what is this? These people have got no idea about what my experience has actually been like – we're working at a completely different level here. Then what really made it for me, what settled it for me, was that one of the group leaders that I knew fairly well by that time, rang me up one day and said, 'I've got somebody in my flat and she's very distressed and I think she's schizophrenic, can you advise me what to do?'. And I thought, hang on a second,

DOI: 10.4324/9781003636434-32

you know [laughs] I'm supposed to be one of your customers, so to speak, one of the people that you're helping, and you're ringing me up asking me how to cope with someone with schizophrenia! And I thought, no, I can't go along with this, it's clear that some of these people don't appear to have the knowledge, basically, to make this a safe place. So, I got out of it after that. I mean, I think at that kind of event, but also in other situations, if people aren't familiar with the experience of using mental health services, using acute wards, using asylums, being given ECT against your will, if you're not familiar with all that negative experience, then it does separate us out, and it does make it difficult. Because I think that, at a certain point, your life experience becomes very different from the general life experience, so you're not just working on your problems, you're working on the problems that the psychiatric system has engineered while trying to help you.

2.22

'WORKING WITH CHILDREN'
[*Testimony* 2000]

Basically, after I left the therapeutic community, what I was trying to do was to work, and possibly develop some kind of career working with children, at the same time as having periodic readmissions into psychiatric hospital. I'd already studied pre-school work. I got a diploma for working with pre-school children before I left the therapeutic community and I started working with children. At one point, I was working with teenagers on adventure playgrounds, but I wasn't tough enough for that, I wasn't enough of an authority figure, so then I concentrated on working with pre-school children and worked in various different places. What happened in the end, towards the end of the seventies, was that basically my psychiatrist, and the caring team, decided that they were going to withdraw their approval for me to go on working with children because I was having crises and they believed it was due to working with children. So, I had to give up working with children, because I couldn't really go on getting work unless I had the backing of my psychiatrist to give me references and support.

I then found work in the book trade for John Menzies and I ended up working for them for about three years in a couple of their shops. In1981, I left John Menzies and I spent the next couple of years doing bits and pieces of jobs.

I moved to Cricklewood in 1983 and I suppose around about that time I decided to give up trying to be a career person and to do what I want to do, and one of the things that I'd always wanted to do, I suppose, was to try to explain to people that they've got it wrong about what so-called mental illness was like, and what it was like to use mental health services. This had always been something that I'd felt strongly about that people really didn't understand what it was like, what our experience was like. And so I decided that I was going to try to get involved in doing something along those lines and I got involved with a MIND association in Camden and then about the same time I started to get involved in the two or three survivor organizations that were then existing in London, the British Network for Alternatives to Psychiatry and the Campaign Against Psychiatric Oppression and that led to setting up other organizations, in particular Survivors Speak Out.

However, one of the important things when I moved to Cricklewood in 1983 was that the psychiatric team that I was in contact with, the new team, they basically

DOI: 10.4324/9781003636434-33

said we'll do all we can to help you get back to working with children. I kind of managed to rehabilitate myself basically to work with children again and for a while until the end of the 1980s, from say 1983 to 1989, I was sort of combining work with service user groups, planning to set up user action groups, with working with children. I started doing voluntary work with children, and then started working for an agency working with children. Until about 1989, I was working with the agency and also doing this work with service user groups at the same time. And then from about 1990 onwards, I started working freelance, earning money as a freelance mental health trainer.

I think I've been very lucky actually. I'd been a revolving door patient if you like, I've been in ten different psychiatric hospitals in the last 30 odd years, I've had 20 something like admissions, but despite that, I've actually been able to work most of the time when I've not been in hospital, and I've actually been able to do things that I quite value doing. OK there have been periods when I've been doing shit jobs, if you like, cleaning, domestic cleaning and industrial temping, all that kind of thing, but I've also worked for ten or fifteen years with preschool children which I think, in a way, is remarkable, that a man with a psychotic illness, a major psychotic illness, has been able to work with preschool children for fifteen years and I've been lucky because I really loved doing it.

Part 3

A QUEST FOR LIBERATION, 2000–2022

3.00

INTRODUCTION TO PART 3, 'A QUEST FOR LIBERATION', 2000–2022

As we saw earlier, Mary Nettle extols a form of leadership that holds it all together by embracing diversity in all senses [2.00]. This is exactly what Peter tries to achieve in an unwavering quest for liberation that is, above all, an ethical undertaking in which, all along the line, he tries to highlight the human significance of what is being proposed or done, to ask what is humanly wrong or wanting, is being humanly overlooked or omitted or denied by the dominant powers, and to identify, and secure, viable spaces for self-discovery [3.06] and for care [3.12]. How are service users regarded and treated as human beings? What compromises and indignities are being enforced on the integrity of the human being or individual agent? How must the service user now imagine herself as a human being? The achievements of survivor action are certainly to be celebrated but every day brings new questions and challenges [3.11]. The survivor critique must meet the challenges of a socio-political system founded on prejudices and misunderstandings of people diagnosed with so-called mental disorders [3.15].

Peter evinces a compelling sense of the depth and complexity of human beings, uttering calls for dialogue, and a search for the understanding of another's distress through authentic engagement, that are only rarely, or imperfectly, reciprocated by his interlocutors. Finding himself yet again in solitary confinement in a bare room in his underpants, he ponders how to salvage a caring imagination that might remedy these conditions [3.12]. The experience of being abandoned in solitary confinement brings into focus questions and feelings that someone in authority should be facing up to [3.13].

How to secure the conditions in which acutely ill, or distressed, people may be supported in a caring, trusting environment [3.05]? Peter is heavily invested in, and committed to, a critical caring imagination that will fasten on the difference, frequently blurred and difficult to distinguish, between genuinely helping the distressed and moulding them for roles as the disempowered. In Peter's estimation, this is the deception that psychiatry frequently perpetrates [3.15]. He is all the time pinpointing, and trying to winkle out, instances where the caring imagination

DOI: 10.4324/9781003636434-35

has gone missing, into hiding or is simply unavailable. Acknowledging the huge importance of advocacy, he leans towards an understanding of advocacy grounded in the critical but invariably vulnerable relationship between advocate and partner [3.07].

A determined non-smoker, he succeeds in keeping his curiosity and spirit of enquiry alive under challenging conditions in a psychiatric hospital day room amidst a thick pallor of smoke and the constant background sound of the television where doing nothing, smoking heavily and sleeping are the norm [3.08]. Though stopping short of recommending that it be banned, he clarifies and underlines through his own experience the status of ECT as a demeaning form of treatment [3.09]. Psychiatry always looks to undermine the competence of survivors, alleging that they do not know what is best for them. Contrary to the presumptions and prejudices of psychiatric experts, Peter maintains that people with mental health problems have access to an ethical knowledge through their experience and suffering. For the most part they know what is good for them and also what good itself is [3.14]. In 3.14 Peter is being asked to take a stand on a proposition. This may be an unfamiliar term to some readers and here it means argument or claim. He maintains a complex position over medications, accepting them in some measure but all the time questioning their benefits and effects on his overall health. Being involved in survivor action has not stopped him going into mental hospitals [3.11] but a life of intermittent crises and hospitalisations is preferable to a condition of being permanently dumbed down [3.10]. The guiding criterion here is feeling alive and being able to create.

Towards the end of his life, Peter acknowledges that the survivor movement may now have lost its critical edge and been co-opted into the mental health system. However, in the emergence of Mad Studies he can identify a survivor-controlled initiative that may provide a critique of psychiatry, rekindle the critical questions and concerns he has long been pursuing, and seek to build alternatives to psychiatry (Beresford & Russo, 2023; see also Warren, 2024). The quest goes on.

References

Beresford, Peter & Russo, Jasna eds (2023) *Routledge International Handbook of Mad Studies* (London: Routledge).

Warren, Sasha (2024) *Storming Bedlam: Madness, Utopia and Revolt* (London: Common Notions).

3.01

'COMING OUT OF THE CLOSET'
[*Testimony* 2000]

I suppose the big thing for me, leaving aside whatever may have been achieved or not by service user organisations that I'd been attached with, is that I was doing something that used my experience in a positive way. Up until the early 1980s, basically, I had part of my life which was totally hidden away, and never spoken of, or spoken of very little. After the early 1980s, I was actually using that part of my life in a positive and constructive way and actually ended up now kind of earning my living by using my personal experience to teach other people. And that, I mean, that's just extremely liberating, and it made me feel a lot different about myself, that I've actually been able to take that experience out of a cupboard and actually look at it and use it in a completely different way than when I was looking at it prior to that.

I mean, that's not to say I haven't got any more problems, but it means that the fact that I've got problems seems much different to me now than it would have done before I started coming out, so to say. So, it's a privilege in a way to have been able to have had the opportunity to do that, I mean I think I've been very lucky actually. I'd been a revolving door patient if you like, I've been in ten different psychiatric hospitals in the last 30 odd years, I've had 20 something like admissions, but despite that, I've actually been able to work most of the time when I've not been in hospital, and I've actually been able to do things that I quite value doing. And then I've been able, in the last fifteen years, to actually use my experience of mental distress, and of using mental health services, in a positive way as well, so I've been very very lucky, particularly when you think that a large number of people with a similar diagnosis to mine and with a similar history of using mental health services, never never work and so, you know, I've been fortunate.

And then, of course, being involved in the service user survivor movement has just meant that I've met tremendous people, you know, really tremendous people and that, I suppose, has been the best part. I've met people who have got very similar experiences to mine, people who are thought by the majority of society to be in the dustbin, to be extremely strange, to be extremely frightening, in actual fact these people I've met, that I know, and are friends of mine, are great people and some of them have made a really good contribution to the understanding of

DOI: 10.4324/9781003636434-36

mental illness and mental distress, mental health problems, whatever you want to call it. And that, in a way, has been very invigorating for me to actually be part of. I suppose it's part of coming out of the closet really, part of a group of people coming out of the closet in historical terms, and that just happens to have coincided with my lifetime and I think I'm very fortunate because, you know, 50 years ago, if I'd been born 50 years earlier, I would never have been a revolving door patient, I would never have got out of the asylum, I would have gone into the asylum and I would have stayed there and that would have been it, it would have been a full stop basically, as far as my life is concerned.

I do feel I'm still a survivor. If someone was to ask me, how do you define yourself in terms of this experience that we're discussing, I think I'd still say that I'm a mental health system survivor, you know. I mean, that implies that I am surviving, rather than that I feel I've survived and it's over. I think I shall go on surviving. I do feel that while, on the one hand, the psychiatric system the asylum, mental health services in the community, and all the rest of it have helped and supported me, but in the end they don't meet my needs, and haven't met my needs over the course of 30 odd years, so that when I look back at it, I'm still surviving a system, an obstacle course, that I know isn't going to meet my needs and I think that's one of the difficulties, when you have to use a system, when you're dependent on a system over a long period of time, and when you actually know that system, because of the way it's set up, cannot meet your needs but that actually puts you in an invidious situation.

I feel, I suppose, as a revolving door patient, if that's what I am, I feel that mental health services have actually been quite good at getting me through crises, I mean I've gone from six months admissions to six weeks admissions, and that basically in terms of getting me up off my knees, and out on the street again, the acute ward does quite well, but what it doesn't do is help me prevent these things happening. Until recent years, it hasn't appeared to be interested in that at all, and it doesn't actually help me to come to terms with my experience. Not only my psychotic experience, which it doesn't appear to be interested in, but also my experience of being a mental health service user, being mentally ill in the eyes of society, and what does it mean in terms of who I am, and who I might become, and that seems to be the big problem with psychiatry. It's like a polo mint, there's a big hole in the middle. And so, ultimately, that is why I would say that I'm a survivor. I mean, I'm very glad that I'm still around 33 years after entering the mental health system and I think if it hadn't been for some of the help I've got there, I wouldn't be alive but, ultimately, I don't think the system is working for me, or for other people, in the way that it could do and that's why, whatever other people say, I am still a survivor of the mental health system.

3.02

'CONTROL IN THE COMMUNITY' BY PETER CAMPBELL, 12TH SEPTEMBER 2000

The balance between care and control has been a major theme in the history of mental health services. In the early nineteenth century, there was a strong belief that madness had to be 'tamed' or broken to uphold reason. When the first asylums were built, they were partly a genuine attempt to create therapeutic environments and partly containers for a group of people who were seen to have no place in a new industrialised society.

These tensions grew worse. The number of asylum inmates increased rapidly. There were no cures available. The medications and other physical treatments used had a strong flavour of control. By the early 20th century, the asylum system looked like a vast holding operation. The heroic period of experimentation starting in the 1920s that led to the development of coma and shock therapies and psycho-surgery altered this pessimistic prospect and gave the impression that mental health services could, after all, change people's lives as well as control them.

But this dilemma did not go away – even after the introduction of major tranquillisers and other psychiatric drugs, arguably the most important 20th century development in care and treatment. Instead, the problem became more complex as care and control began to shift out of the controlled environment of the asylum to the less certain and riskier territories of the community.

It is possible to see mental health services as acting, inadvertently or by design, as an agent of social control. History could support this view. It was one of the entry points to service user action in the early 1980s. Psychiatry certainly seems to control a lot of individuals. But, the dividing line between care and control may not always be clear cut and it may not just be people with a mental illness diagnosis that are vulnerable.

The particular difficulty for us is that we are traditionally seen as unaware of our own best interests and therefore at risk of coming under the control of experts who know what is best for us better than we do. This is fine as long as our goals and their goals coincide reasonably well – and it could be that this has become more likely in the last 30 years. But care, based on our wants, still frequently slips into control based on what professionals say we really need. And the Mental Health Act, based around a denial of our right to control our own bodies, stands in the background – a framework encouraging control.

DOI: 10.4324/9781003636434-37

The period since the 1983 Mental Health Act has seen continuing concern – by governments, service providers, service users and latterly society itself – over the amount of control that should be exercised over people with a mental illness diagnosis in the community. Compliance with care and treatment, particularly drug treatments, has become a key issue. Although the government has made it clear that they will include a community treatment order in any new Mental Health Act, the arguments are not yet resolved.

One argument in defence of a community treatment power is that it enables the recipient to be treated in the least restrictive setting. In this view, it is less controlling than an order that makes someone spend time on an acute ward. While this seems a reasonable point, it is worth wondering what sort of life you will lead on a community order – taking medication against your will, forced to attend day centres, work programmes, counselling. Certainly, a restricted daily life.

Another argument is that mental health professionals are well skilled in working within a compulsory framework. Acquiring more power over service users will not damage their relationships. This viewpoint (usually proposed by professionals) is based on a rather more generous assessment of their usual handling of compulsory powers than many service users might make. But it is also influenced by the fact that, in the general run of things, mental health professionals expect their relationships to service users to be relationships where they are in control. More power for the powerful is always something they can handle.

The values motivating the mental health services are vital in developing a better balance between care and control. The emergence of compliance as a key goal is not simply linked to closer concern with the best interests of service useless but also comes from mental health professionals picking up, or being pressured to pick up, the social control function of services. While achieving a calmer settlement between people with a mental illness and society may be a legitimate aim, the danger is that compliance cannot provide the degree of social control government expects and in the meanwhile the character of services deteriorates in the hands of professionals desensitised to what distinguishes care from control.

3.03

'SURVIVING SOCIAL INCLUSION'
(c 2000) BY PETER CAMPBELL
[Excerpted]

'Health and Social Services should promote mental health for all, work with indi-viduals and communities, combat discrimination against groups with mental health problems and promote their social inclusion'.
Standard One of the National Service Framework

Introduction: where do I belong?

Napsbury hospital closed in the summer of 1999. Not an event of huge importance in the scale of things but of personal significance for me. I had been using Naps-bury regularly since 1984. It was 'my bin'. Its closure meant the destruction of a familiar if not much-loved place of refuge.

But Napsbury Hospital was never my home. Nor were any of the other units and asylums I ended up in over the last 30 years. Like many of my generation of long-term service users, I never spent years in any one hospital. Although I have spent four or five years in asylums of one kind or another, I have never belonged to the asylum. In many senses, North West London has been my home over the last 20 years. Settling where I now live after a long period on the bed-sit circuit was one of the most significant developments in my life. But on what terms do I, the holder of a mental illness ticket, belong in my 'home' community? On terms of self-imposed secrecy to be honest. I once shared a house with three others, got admitted twice in two years, and mental illness was never mentioned. That was in the 1970s, but even now, while I am open and confident with fellow survivors, I keep a plausible story up my sleeve for the football terraces or the café.

And we have good reason to be cautious. A few years ago, I had an argument with the couple who lived downstairs. At its climax the man shouted out: 'We all know about you. You're a nutter. You've got no rights round here.' I have friends who were driven out of their homes because they were seen to be 'nutters'. It isn't just a thing of the past. In the mid-1980s, when service user action was just starting,

In: *This is Madness Too: Critical Perspectives on Mental Health*, Craig Newness, Guy Holmes & Cail-zie Dunn eds (PCCS Book, 2001)

DOI: 10.4324/9781003636434-38

I agreed to be photographed in my flat by the local newspaper to publicise a new group. For all the activity and the brave rhetoric of the last fifteen years, there is no way I would stand up for that job today.

I have been fortunate in that at the point when I was running out of ideas as to how to fit into a conventional career and lifestyle and be a 'serial lunatic' at the same time, the identity of mental patient began to open out and – through the service user/survivor movement – I found some positive places where I belonged. Nevertheless, it is easy to overestimate what is going on inside, and on the fringes, of the mental health services and to believe that the fact that people with a diagnosis of psychotic illness are being jetted out to conferences in Frankfurt or Japan has a wider significance. Society's response to the 'community mental patient' is quite uncertain (Barham, 1997). Our acceptance, along with other disabled people, is provisional not definite. We may not be returning to crude measures to include us out – 'euthanasia' programmes, compulsory sterilisation, although we know all about that now. But how far society is prepared to go to include us in? That is a different matter.

Social inclusion: a controlling contract?

The promise of social inclusion is not a new one. General or specific, spoken or implied, it has drifted over the field of mental health services for the best part of the last 40 years. The gap between the promise and the reality, for people who had since the 1960s been present in the community if not part of it, was one of the basic, if less emphasised, reasons for the growth in service user/survivor action. But the image and reality of inclusion does not only have resonance for service users. But a certain point in the last 20 years – and the NHS and Community Care Act 1990 may be some kind of a marker – large parts of society woke up to the fact that 'the mentally ill' were indeed no longer 'there' but 'here'. The house on the hill with its long boundary walls, gate house and tower could no longer continue to be the symbolic or actual container for this group. It was the street corners and public libraries now. And, while at one level, de facto inclusion was sanctioned by society, at another what society was really interested in was not inclusion but control.

It is certainly welcome to see the social and political context of mental health services acknowledged in the NSF Standard One. The commitments to combat discrimination and promote social inclusion are helpful. But on what basis is inclusion to be offered to people with a mental illness diagnosis? To what extent do we remain a special group in society, whose full participation is conditional on particular behaviour?

These difficulties may not be unique to people with a mental illness diagnosis. Disabled people and other groups share them to some extent. But we face the particular difficulty that, of all disabled people, we are the ones most likely to be thought both unaware of our best interests and a direct threat to society. These two perceptions make it particularly easy for unusual interventions to be attached to our lifestyles and our participation kept out on the margins.

Service users/survivors have probably never been in a strong position to negotiate anything with society. This is not being helped by a deepening gulf that has grown up in recent years between who service users think they are, and might become, and what the government, the media and society think. While many mental health workers clearly believe that people with a mental illness diagnosis have a positive contribution to make, in reality they have had to witness a government approach focused in an essentially negative vision (Campbell, 1999) [−].

Continually returning to the longstanding negative perceptions about mad persons must jeopardise the chances of meaningful inclusion. Even if you add on at the end that only a small percentage actually fulfil the stereotypes. Social inclusion needs to be based on a positive vision, a belief that the newly included will bring something valuable, not that if we watch them closely enough then they probably won't mess up. There are positive foundations for social inclusion and some of these have been indicated by service user/survivor organisations: equal value, equal opportunities, inclusive diversity, the chance to contribute, the chance to opt out, rights, tolerance of difference (Craine, 1998). But they coexist with equally compelling factors like concepts of risk and dangerousness, compliance with treatment and care plans. The challenge for service user/survivor organisations is to ensure that social inclusion remains an opportunity for us and not a chance to patch the fences because we made it back to town.

The idea of citizenship as a type of contract where rights are linked to, and grounded in, responsibilities is currently influential. This development may be of uncertain benefit to a conspicuously powerless group like mental health service users, particularly if it starts to impinge on aspects of their service use. Marjorie Wallace of SANE has written: '… essentially care in the community is a "contract" agreed with mentally ill people, balancing their rights against their responsibilities to live within certain rules necessary for the well-being and peace of mind of others' (Wallace, 1999). Although give and take is necessary for any community inclusion, one must wonder in the current climate, how many and what kind of rules 'mentally ill people' would have to satisfy to establish 'the well-being and peace of mind of others'. More than observing the law of the land, one imagines.

In the above scenario, it does not seem too fanciful to suggest that the written care plan may play an increasingly significant role. And not just for those on compulsory orders. Society, learning from mental health workers, invests tremendous significance in people with a mental illness diagnosis 'taking their treatments'. What better symbol of that than when the individual 'signs up', showing their willingness to be 'controlled', their capacity to be 'in control'. It would not take very much – indeed it is probably already happening – for the care plan (introduced 1991) to slide from being an outline of desired interventions to an agreement to comply. With the latter emphasis it could become a reliable passport to inclusion, carrying the mental health services' dual imperatives – to care for and control – out into society.

The terms for people's inclusion in mental health services, for their inclusion in society and the links between the two, need open discussion. It may be unrealistic to expect that long-disadvantaged groups can be included into society on an equal basis. But it seems self-defeating to reinforce or introduce new inequalities into the mechanics of inclusion. The current contract available to people with a mental illness diagnosis – both as citizens and as service users – appears to be linked to a vision of our essentially anti-social contribution and to the need for compliance. This sort of deal may reassure society and keep the mental health system ticking over. Whether it is a suitable basis for the liberation of community mental patients remains to be seen.

Conclusion

[−] Service user survivor groups face practical difficulties in effectively communicating with the public. The public are an unfamiliar audience and groups may have to learn different languages and techniques to those that have proved successful within mental health services. But the greater difficulties may lie in a struggle over the terms of inclusion, the balance of rights and responsibilities, and who controls the messages that go out concerning people with a mental illness diagnosis. If groups are to take serious action to change public behaviour (and there is evidence that direct experience can be effective in altering attitudes), they must create and contribute to a debate on what mental health education is about rather than be illustrative material in an expert consensus. They must consider setting up specialist public education groups. They must hold to their own vision of social inclusion.

Equal access to work opportunities, civil rights legislation, a more accurate and sensitive mass media are all desirable aspects of the enthusiasm for social inclusion. But they do not automatically lead to a feeling of belonging. Whatever happens in the next few years, people with a mental illness diagnosis will be hiding their psychiatric histories in their left shoe for some time yet. In the meantime, service user/survivor activists and others should bear in mind that while inclusion on the right basis could be liberating, inclusion on the wrong basis could prove as painful as exclusion in the old asylums.

References

Barham, P. (1997) *Closing the Asylum: The Mental Patient in Modern Society*. London: Penguin Books.

Campbell, P. (1999) 'The Service User/Survivor Movement', in: Newnes, C., Holmes, G., & Dunn, C., eds. *This Is Madness: A Critical Look at Psychiatry and the Future of Mental Health Services*. Ross- on-Wye: PCCS Books.

Craine, S. (1998) *Shrink Resistant: The Survivor Movement and the Survivor Perspective*. US Network Working Papers, Exchange & Change.

Wallace, M. (1999) Letter on community care in *The Independent*, Friday 19 November 1999.

3.04

'DISCHARGED' [*Testimony* 2000]

'After you come out of hospital what's it like picking up from where you left off?'

'Well, it gets increasingly difficult, I think, and that's partly to do with getting older. Twenty years ago, or fifteen years ago, I could kind of go through that process and recover fairly quickly, and now I think it takes me much longer, maybe six months, to fully recover after I've been discharged. Most people in the mental health services never consider how you settle back into the community that you live in after you've exited that community in a very dramatic way. If you've drawn attention to yourself, you've made a big scene of some kind, you disappear for six weeks and you suddenly reappear, how do you actually reestablish your credibility, and how do you get to feel OK about people who must know, to some degree or other, what's going on?

I'm more used to that than I used to be but it's still a problem, a big problem and a worry, and by and large I've never been asked what I feel about being discharged and going back, it's just, you know, it's just assumed that I'm competent to do it. One of the things that is a major problem for me at the time is that I usually trash my flat to some degree. I'm a very tidy person normally but I will disrupt things. I won't smash things up, but I'll disrupt things, so usually there's a lot of clearing, cleaning, and tidying to be done when I'm discharged and that is quite difficult. You spend the first two days after discharge cleaning up your place, when your energy levels haven't really been restored.'

DOI: 10.4324/9781003636434-39

3.05

'A BARREN EXPERIENCE' (A CRISIS ADMISSION) BY 'NIALL' (2001) *Mental Health Today*, September 2001

I have just spent the last part of June and the first part of July as an in-patient in a psychiatric unit. Although I have in the past been a regular recipient of admission ward care, there were two major changes since my last crisis that greatly affected the service I received. One was that the unit was brand new, being purpose built to replace wards in the old hospital outside the city. The other was that since my previous last admission I have acquired a significant hearing impairment.

The physical environment was excellent: no nicotine-stained ceilings, no punctured armchairs. Generally, the ward was bright, clean and pleasant to use, not at all like some older city units I have seen. Although it was cramped everyone had their own room and, while there were no spacious gardens, decent shops were five minutes walk away rather than a 20-minute bus ride. I spent some of the two final weeks of my admission-once I was allowed off the ward- looking for second-hand paperbacks in the local thrift shops.

The ward itself was cross-shaped with the nursing office at the centre where the four short corridors converged. For reasons not known, the patients' telephone was also situated there, opposite six always-occupied chairs. It was the most unprivate place possible. The telephone's location meant that calls were few and always short – which perhaps explains its positioning.

Hearing loss

Problems around my hearing were an important feature of my stay. The unit almost completely lacked 'deaf awareness'. The police had delivered me to the ward with no shoes, no glasses, no hearing aids. I was distressed, confused and angry. No one thought of communicating through writing until a friend came to see me three days later. My flat keys were in security. The friend told me no one seemed particularly concerned that if the keys were not retrieved the next day (a Friday, security being closed over the weekend) I would be without these essentials until Monday at the earliest. Eventually, I had to write a letter authorising her use of my keys. It is hard not to feel staff lack flexibility and imagination when faced by unusual difficulties.

 DOI: 10.4324/9781003636434-40

Things got better once I recovered my hearing aids–but not much. In the ward round I was seated furthest from the consultant, who shouted at me rather than inviting me to move closer. Most of the nurses made no special effort to adapt to my difficulties. The noise level on the ward was so high–two of the patients communicated almost entirely through shouting–that my ears hurt inside. In the end I kept my hearing aids in but turned off for 60 to 70% of the time I spent in social settings, blocking sound completely. I could not watch TV or hear radio in the communal areas because of background noise.

Occupational therapy was difficult but at least it was quieter. My feeling of isolation, always strong when I am working to get out of psychiatric hospital, was very much worse this time. I hardly had a conversation with another in-patient which, as others who have been in psychiatric hospital will know, makes the journey really sticky.

The first ten days were not easy and were made more difficult because I had arrived via a section 136. I had been placed in solitary confinement in a police cell (again) awaiting assessment. I remain convinced this practice should simply be outlawed. It multiplied my distress several times. I may be partial but I cannot conceive of many human beings who would not be paranoid and angry after such treatment. I was certainly shocked, even traumatised.

Containment

It was no surprise to me that medication created difficulties. I suffered several extra-pyramidal effects: stiffening of posture, joints etc. My friend noticed this on the Thursday and told me to tell staff. I didn't and a nurse only noted it on the Sunday. I was given an intramuscular injection of something within half an hour and the negative effects immediately subsided. A mental health system survivor identified after just 20 minutes something noticed by only one out of some 16 staff who had been with me on eight-hour shifts for nearly a week.

I'm not suggesting that staff were incompetent. But the average level of skills and knowledge among the nurses did not appear very high. They were working under stress. The ward was certainly 'active'. The outer door was locked most of the time. One or two nurses looked exhausted and stressed out. I felt one or two were working within themselves to avoid stresses. There was a lot of close observation, both mobile and from chairs outside individuals' rooms. Nursing seemed dominated by supervision and containment and, for senior nurses, paperwork in the office. Nothing new there, then.

One Sunday I asked a nurse four times for time to talk. No success. The next day, immediately following a positive phone call from a friend, I shouted: 'Yes, I'm really going to get out of this place'. Within 30 seconds two large male nurses were on either side of me, wanting to know what was up. If I did something antisocial, I was noticed, but not otherwise. Eventually I gave up and worked my passage solo.

Two nurses were the great exception to this rule. One senior, one junior, both of them knew me from before this admission–the senior for almost 15 years. They were the saving grace. Individually kind and interested in what I had been doing with my life, they helped me discover I can, despite my hearing loss, still appreciate a lot of music (something I had not confronted since a disastrous start three years ago). Through their encouragement and the loan of a cassette radio and a relaxation tape, they did me a great service.

A not insignificant victory was that my section was rescinded after two weeks once I had proved myself by going down to my flat and coming back promptly. This was the first time in about a dozen detentions over the years that I have been taken off a section while still in hospital. It may not seem much but it meant a lot for my dignity and self-esteem. Moreover, I felt it was some payback for all those occasions when everyone knew I was competent and co-operating but my requests to be taken off the section were refused. Many mental health workers think they are good at using the Mental Health Act. I do not agree.

One of the themes of crisis and recovery for me is the theme of fall and redemption. While I feel I am a failure, at a deep level I enjoy the task of return and the period of heightened awareness that goes with it. Eating in a café, buying a damaged Star Trek novel, schooling myself to read again–all have a special feel as in childhood. June and July 2001 were no different in this respect and I'm grateful for that, from wherever it comes. But in other ways the journey was a barren experience for me. Acute wards no longer foster people's latent humanity. Crisis houses and home treatment may or may not do so. It is possible that the difficulties of treating acutely ill people in a caring, trusting environment cannot be resolved and that lowering rather than raising my expectations might be more realistic, for the foreseeable future at least.

3.06

"IT'S NOT THE REAL YOU."
[Draft March 2001 for *OpenMind*]

Most long-term recipients will have a personal list of professional catch phrases that have punctuated their lives within services. Stock sentiments that contain distress and dissent, establish boundaries, oil the wheels of the caring machine, moving people on from drugs trolley to ward round, from office door to yet another session of TV watching.

Near the top of my own list comes "It's not the real you….", a phrase that, in exactly this, or a very similar form has pursued me through the greater part of my career as a recipient. Whatever the intentions behind its use (and it is the nature of such catch phrases to harbor complex intentions), "It's not the real you…." has always been able to get right under my skin. On one level, it is the absurdity of people who have never met me until the evening I was brought onto the ward, feeling they can get away with such sweeping judgements. The fact that there is a box file of information about "the real me" in the nursing office written by professionals with whom I have never had a cup of tea only makes the situation worse. Any idea that professional carers know me better than I do myself – an extremely dangerous proposition, in my opinion – has to be based on more than this.

But the phrase also conveys separation and denial. "It's not the real you…" closes down (for whatever reason) areas of perception, experience, dissent. And, although in traditional societies, the fact that this material is associated with the unreal might give it positive value, in contemporary British society that connection can only be negative. Edmund Podvoll writes about "asylum mind" and its most subtle manifestation, "the silence that humiliates" – a deliberate rift between doctor and patient (1). I see "It's not the real you…" as an example of the general withdrawal of mental health workers from aspects of my life. A withdrawal which, in the context of the acute ward, is both tangible (I am forced to share space with an absence) and judgemental (at some point my idea of "the real me" and their idea of "the real you" is going to have to coincide enough for me to get back to my own place).

But this does not just concern mental health workers. A number of my family and loved ones have adopted versions of the "It's not the real you…" approach over the years to help explain situations, and to minimize my responsibility for things

DOI: 10.4324/9781003636434-41

I have said or done during crises. Although they have usually had a greater understanding of who I am, and much less opportunity to let their judgements invade my life, ultimately they are also categorizing and evaluating my actions, relegating some to a second or third division of significance.

And, of course, I am involved in something similar myself. Like many people with a mental illness diagnosis, identity is a living issue for me. Ever since I was catapulted from the status of undergraduate scholar to that of long-term mental patient, questions about "who am I now?" and "what was going on back there?" have been central. Within this exploration, behaviour that I find problematic has played a significant part. The fact that, at a time when I was working with preschool children, I struck an approved social worker and on occasions was sufficiently "challenging" to be forcibly injected or thrown into solitary confinement was a major dilemma. One to which mental health workers were largely insensitive. In the end, I have resorted to a process of distancing from these actions that advances a little way down the ladder of "It's not the real you…", by seeing them as uncharacteristic, but stops well short of any assertion that they are not a part of who I am. While patience and gentleness have been important aspects of my self-image, I do not see anger and aggression as diseases foreign to my nature.

The struggle of people with a mental illness diagnosis over who they really are is not simply about disagreements over what perceptions, experiences, and actions are problematic. It also concerns how individuals can place and value characteristics they acknowledge as problems. In this undertaking, one major difficulty is that many service recipients want to integrate problem aspects into themselves, and develop some positive value for them, while many service providers (and others) want us to get rid of them altogether. So, while I have never met a recipient on an acute ward who has said "I am going straight out there to get mad again", I have met a large number who clearly feel, as I do, that their madness (however they define it) is essential to them. A problem that we must address – but not just in narrow terms of denigration and destruction.

I am not looking to mental health workers for active help in discovering or creating "the real me", although they may be successfully assisting others in this regard. But I would like them to be sensitive to the huge negative impact they may be having on service users' attempts to forge positive identities. One of the most damaging features of "It's not the real you…" judgements is that their main target is psychotic actions, thoughts, and perceptions. The categorical dismissal of this area of experience (from which mental health services are only starting to emerge) is then closely linked with concepts like insight, unpredictability, and best interests to create a web invalidating the worlds of many people who experience mental distress. Our trouble is not that we have desirable and less desirable characteristics but that we are judged to have too much of the unreal in us.

Although professional expertise has helped me over the years, it's power to possess and shut out should never be underestimated. I remember first reading that 2 to 3% of the population hear voices and that two-thirds of them never become psychiatric patients. I remember thinking "But, of course!" I had always known where the horizon was, but the experts scrambled my vision.

In recent years, I believe it has become more possible for people with a mental illness diagnosis to explore and express who they really are. But I wouldn't make any great claims about progress or underestimate the obstacles to further change. I have been lucky to be around when the identities (and job opportunities) available to some community mental patients have opened up a little. Yet these developments may not have touched the majority, and, while I now have a better sense of a positive "real me", I am more careful how I express this than I was ten years ago. Although it is unfashionable to talk of psychiatric oppression nowadays, society keeps a steady grip on who I am allowed to be.

Moreover, the "real/unreal" you division is connected to the belief that there are right and wrong types of distress and right and wrong ways of expressing distress and that somehow I have been getting it fundamentally wrong. This sense of not just doing it wrong but of "being in the wrong" is difficult to shake off. It is closely related to what the philosopher Charles Taylor has identified as an individual person's need to be properly orientated to the good and is one of the major unstated targets of all service user/survivor action (2). Individually and collectively, we are staking out new territory on which we can stand.

In the early nineteenth century psychiatrists like John Haslam asserted that the dividing line between madness and sanity was fixed and clear cut (3). Now we are not so certain. This does not mean that we have stopped drawing lines across the lives of people with a mental illness diagnosis, putting aspects above and below, within and outside the divisions. Nor that some experiences, although open to consideration, are not deemed wrong, functionally and morally. Action by mental health service recipients is undermining some of this. But the struggle remains, not just to create better mental health services, but to secure a space for self-discovery.

References

1. Podvoll, E. (1990) *The Seduction of Madness* (Century).
2. Taylor, C. (1989) *Sources of the Self* (Cambridge University Press).
3. Haslam, J. (1988) *Illustrations of Madness*, Roy Porter ed. (Routledge).

3.07

'AN OUTLINE HISTORY OF MENTAL HEALTH ADVOCACY IN ENGLAND'

Any attempt at an account of mental health advocacy in England should begin with the definition of advocacy. This is not easy. There have been numerous descriptions over the last 30 years, and these can lead to confusion. One approach is to look at advocacy in a broad sense. Thus, a wide range of activities involving different actions and skills can be included: committee work, lobbying and campaigning, education. In the 1980s, Mind even described the provision of good hostels, housing, day centres etc. as 'exemplary advocacy'. On the other hand, there is a narrower approach focusing on the individual relationship between an advocate and a partner. This is the way I prefer to see advocacy. To me, it is not so much about working, often with groups of people, to achieve general goals at some point in the future, as a relationship where an individual seeks to secure the wants of an individual/individuals in the immediate future. It involves a set of particular skills that are quite different from campaigning and lobbying etc.

Advocacy is not a new concept. The idea of speaking and acting for someone who has difficulty in doing so for her/himself goes back for centuries. It may not be too fanciful to think of the Good Samaritan as an early advocate. But advocacy that gives significant control to the partner involved in the process is a more recent development. For most of the last 200 years mental health advocacy has been paternalistic and the process (if not the outcome) cannot be described as empowering. People diagnosed as mentally ill have been considered as incompetent, unable to judge what was in their best interests, prevented by their illness even from the ability to give consent. It is only in the last 30 or 40 years that the insight and expertise of service users have begun to be recognized. In this sense, it can be said that empowering advocacy has been a relatively recent development.

Although the nineteenth century can be seen as a classic era of paternalism towards service users, there is one important example of an organization that provided advocacy: The Alleged Lunatics' Friend Society (ALFS) 1845–63. This is

Published in 'The Advocate', February 2004, pp. 9–11, the magazine of the UK Advocacy Network (UKAN) which ceased work around 2010 and were dissolved as a company in 2013.

DOI: 10.4324/9781003636434-42

an exceptional example of advocacy provision and has often been cited as a fore-runner of today's advocacy groups. ALFS was a service user-led organization that included some relatives of current or former asylum inmates and one or two politicians. It was involved in advocacy in the broadest sense but is estimated to have taken up at least 70 individual cases during its lifetime. A great deal of ALFS time and energy was devoted to influencing government and promoting asylum reform through legislation. It believed that people with a mental illness diagnosis should be treated as adults having capability of making decisions for themselves. It proposed (unsuccessfully) that there should be a judicial hearing before admission and asserted that inmates' rights should be posted up in asylums. Alongside such lobbying, ALFS was also involved in education, producing pamphlets and holding (not very well attended) public meetings where former inmates could tell their stories of confinement.

The ALFS had modest success in its work with government. Some of the improvements they suggested led to change only after the group's demise. One historian believes that the organization might have been more effective if its demands had been less radical and its emphasis on the inmates' viewpoint had been less marked – a judgement that may echo the development of survivor action over the last 30 years. Nevertheless, the same historian concedes that ALFS was important in keeping up pressure on the Lunacy Commission and causing a constant reappraisal of policies (Hervey, 1986). The organization also provided much support for individuals and initiated inquiries into the management of numerous asylums.

The historical record does not include many examples of advocacy groups until after the Second World War. For a long period, service users were considered inferior and incapable. Eugenics was popular. In the early 1900s, Winston Churchill declared, 'The unnatural and increasingly rapid growth of the feeble-minded classes, coupled with a steady restriction among all the thrifty, energetic and superior stocks constitutes a race danger. I feel that the source from which the stream of madness is fed should be cut off and sealed up before another year has passed' (letter to Prime Minister Herbert Asquith). When such views are possible, it is impossible for advocacy to flourish.

Positive developments really took shape in the 1970s following the success of civil rights campaigning in the USA. The attitude of mental health workers had also been changing since the 1950s and service users were treated more sensitively. Even so, there were a number of scandals at mental handicap and psychiatric hospitals. Mind began to provide legal advocacy and took a number of cases to the European Court of Human Rights. Rights began to be seen as important as care and the establishment of the Advocacy Alliance in 1981 (mainly focusing on advocacy for people with learning difficulties) helped to bring advocacy into the limelight.

The most important boost for mental health advocacy came with the development of service user/survivor groups. These not only challenged the myth of incompetence but specifically demanded advocacy services. A number of pioneering projects were established. Nottingham Advocacy Group (NAG) that provided patients' councils and individual advocacy was particularly important. Not only was it the first user-led advocacy organization in England but it also was active in spreading the word across England.

In 1992, The United Kingdom Advocacy Network (UKAN) was founded, based in Sheffield. This has been and continues to be a vital organization for promoting mental health advocacy, particularly service-user led advocacy. It has provided leadership and support including training in advocacy skills. Important UKAN publications have been an Advocacy Code of Practice and an Advocacy Reader. Its management committee includes regional representatives from across the UK and its membership includes hundreds of advocacy and service-user action groups. It has played a significant part in the development of advocacy throughout the UK.

These are examples of important grassroots action. What has been the role of government in the growth of advocacy provision? Here, rhetoric has been more prominent than action. Governments have been keen on 'user involvement' since the mid-1980s and this has helped to create a situation where the importance of advocacy can be clearly seen. The need to help people to be involved in their own care and treatment, and to take part in consultation service development, has been recognized. On the other hand, governments have been reluctant to create a right to advocacy and we still do not have this. The Disabled Persons (Services, Consultation and Representation) Act 1986 could have been a major step forward, but the Conservative government refused to implement the most important clauses. After this the right to advocacy was overlooked, only to emerge more recently in the discussions around a new Mental Health Act.

So, we have come to critical moments for mental health advocacy that will decide the future shape of provision. After centuries of the idea, the practice of advocacy has developed rapidly in the last 30 years. Issues of quality and effectiveness are now central. The existence of advocacy is not in question. The nature of advocacy remains in doubt.

The future of advocacy is closely linked to the development of a new Mental Health Act. After appearing lukewarm towards advocacy in the initial stages of consultation, the government seems to have accepted that advocates will have an important role in supporting people compulsorily detained. At the same time, the practice of advocacy will be monitored and standard training programmes set up. Research around good practice is already being undertaken. It is hoped that the quality and effectiveness of the advocacy relationship will improve.

What is not so clear is who will control and provide advocacy projects. It is very possible that service-users, who have played such an important role in bringing advocacy out of the shadows and creating local projects, may be forced to the sidelines. There is already a mixture of organizations involved in provision including voluntary organizations like Mind and Rethink that are not service-user led. These may be seen as more established and reliable than service-user led groups and so dominate the field. It is likely that monitoring and training will become the responsibility of mental health professionals with service users in a subsidiary role.

Does this matter? History suggests that there is a strong tendency for people to do things FOR service users rather than WITH them. Service user organizations have always promoted the self-advocacy principle where the advocacy process is empowering. While it may not be true that only service users can be good advocates, it can certainly be argued that service-user-led projects are likely to be less paternalistic. There is a danger that advocates will become remote and over-professionalized. Maintaining the role of service users in advocacy provision could be the best way of ensuring quality.

Reference

Hervey, N (1986) 'Advocacy or folly: The Alleged Lunatics' Friend Society, 1845–63' *Medical History* 30: 245–75.

3.08

ADAPTED FROM INTERVIEW WITH PETER ABOUT NAPSBURY PSYCHIATRIC HOSPITAL
(*Testimony* 2005, Interviewer Peter Barham)

A lot of the large asylums seem to have very beautiful locations. Quite often they've got very spacious grounds, they're set in nice parts of the landscape and certainly two or three of the asylums that I've been in have that kind of a situation. I think I would say Napsbury is a beautiful place. It's on a slight slope and looks across a shallow valley and up to the horizon there is Shenley which is another psychiatric hospital which I was in briefly and there's also Shenley Tower which is quite nice. Then there are fields in front of the hospital which I think used to belong to a farm which was part of the hospital. I remember one occasion, when I was in Napsbury in the autumn, there were flocks of geese eating in the fields just outside the grounds and I could see them every morning when I got up in the dormitory. I could look out and see the geese out there. So, it's quite a beautiful setting; and some of the trees and shrubs were interesting and they were planted by William Goldring who was also involved in Kew Gardens. Some of the trees are foreign types of trees – I know nothing about that sort of thing – it was very beautiful. There was the main hospital and then villas, villas in the grounds, and loads of lawns and the lawns were always very well kept but I remember being in Napsbury shortly before it closed – I think at the end of the 1990s – and one of the things I noticed were the lawns were no longer being mown properly and that was like an end of an era. But there were large lawns and summer houses in some of the lawns – many of the summer houses were in a bad state of repair by the time I got there in the early 1980s, but you could still sit in them. So, there were probably four or five summer houses, and the lawns were in sections – two or three wards, and lawns outside the wards and then there were some hedges and another series of lawns. I don't know if that was somehow a development of the airing courts – I don't know.

There was a cricket pitch out at the front, and football pitches, and I remember watching the hospital team play London Colney which is the village just outside

DOI: 10.4324/9781003636434-43

Napsbury gates. I watched a few games of football – it was the hospital team, not patients. The grounds were in some way restorative. I found that when I had kind of achieved my freedom to be able to go out of the ward, quite often I would go and sit on the benches round the garden, and I would sit there for maybe an hour or half an hour. I might have done that a couple of times a day. If you were a long stay patient or on one of the rehabilitation wards you might have been part of a gang that would go and help the gardeners.

I remember sometimes in occupational therapy (OT) we would go out and harvest some of the apples and things from the orchards. I mean the orchards were sort of semi derelict, they weren't properly kept, but there had been lots of orchards and also greenhouses which again I remember going to – I'm not quite sure when – probably sometime in the early 1990s, and they again were pretty much derelict as well, and they had supplied loads of flowers to the hospital, vegetables and things as well, but were not fully operating by then. I think in a way, Napsbury was kind of running down by the time I got there in the early 1980s. It was no longer at its peak and things were on the slide, if you like, in terms of facilities. One of the things I remember is in terms of entertainment, in hospitals I was in in the 1970s there used to be quite regular entertainment, like a film in the main hall and quite a lot of dancing and socials – parties on various wards that you could go to, and in Napsbury that seemed to have pretty much gone by the time I was using Napsbury – there weren't dances, there weren't cinema shows, there were still some parties on the wards, but not very big really. All that kind of entertainment side of it had kind of slipped away.

I'm glad to see the asylums have gone for many reasons but I think the setting and the grounds, I kind of miss those. I would say I miss the gardens. I used to go out of the ward and kind of wander round the grounds for a period of time and in a lot of the psychiatric units now, you couldn't really do that. There wouldn't be much point in doing that, apart from buying something from the shops. So yes, what I can say is it certainly helped me to have the gardens, to use the gardens, to be able to walk around, because they're quite extensive so you could have a decent walk around. For me it was a solitary thing. I can't remember going round the grounds with other people. I mean, I would go to the hospital shop, or go along the main corridor of the hospital, with other people and occasionally go up to the shop outside at the hospital gates, but I think going for walks in the garden was a solitary thing for me, it was getting away from the ward, and getting away from people, that was part of it. Yes, it was kind of in a way forgetting that you'd spent hours stuck on a ward with a load of other people! So, you would kind of escape, rather than it being a social activity! I do remember, sometimes in the Summer we would sit out in the bit of garden by the ward I was in, but basically it was a solitary activity.

One of the things I remember, and it's a feature of a lot of asylums, is the corridors, and Napsbury did have long corridors right though the main building and kind of branching off. That was quite gloomy – the floors were always kept polished – that was one thing they always did and there was this machine that used to come along polishing the linoleum, but it was quite gloomy and quite depressing.

I think that that feeling got worse as the hospital was being run down, as a lot of the wards in the main hospital had become empty by then, so you would be walking along these corridors in the evening and it was totally deserted and you got this feeling of this deserted old building. So that was the feature of the big asylums. In the ward itself – usually quite bare and a minimum of furniture, and usually an area with tables in it which is where mealtimes would be, then a day room with lots of armchairs quite often not in very good states of repair, lots of cigarette burns on the floor usually, bare, but kept clean, kept tidy, but fairly bare.

Silver Birch was the admission unit, which was in a villa separate from the main hospital. In Silver Birch you had small dormitory rooms with maybe two or three or three or four beds in it. The dormitories quite often had just a screen as a partition from each other and you would have a locker and a bed and there wasn't a bedside chair, as I remember, and the lockers of course were supposed to be secure, but I think in 37 years of using an asylum I have never come across a locker with a lock. There may be a lock there but there was no key to it. So that was the dormitories.

The bathroom system was you had to get a key to use the bath. It was opened up for you and sometimes there was a shower as well. I wasn't too happy about the lack of privacy in some of the toilet areas, not being able to lock the toilet door and not being sure if you could lock the bathroom door and things like that. And one of the things, you don't have plugs in basins, and it was quite difficult to get hot water. You had to wash under the flowing tap, you can't have a basin full of water. That is pretty standard in those places. I can see safety reasons for not having a plug – because you're going to have spillage and all the rest of it, possibly it's a danger, and you can perhaps self-harm in a basin full of water. But it is a nuisance and certainly in Napsbury the facilities, including the toilet facilities, were kind of Spartan really. There was no soap, you were supposed to provide your own soap. Times have certainly changed. I remember in West Park in the early 1970s working in the hospital stores and taking supplies like soap and things out to the wards. One time in Napsbury in the 1990s, I recall being in the washroom in Silver Birch and a nurse came in and started up a conversation with me. I suddenly noticed that at the same time he was trying to pinch my piece of soap for some task he had to do!

One of the things I remember, this is going off the point a bit, but in terms of getting to be on your own, there weren't enough or any quiet rooms. I remember in Silver Birch there wasn't a quiet room you could use, so I used the toilet – that seemed the only place that was readily available. I might go there every couple of days for the maximum of a quarter of an hour, just to sit there. In later days it was possible to get access to one of the consulting rooms, if you asked them, but that's not a great place to relax either. I've been in hospitals where they have proper quiet rooms with easy chairs, and maybe a radio, but anyway an area where you could be on your own, or with a couple of other people, and relax, but not that many wards in Napsbury had quiet rooms and I remember at one stage they were actually trying to develop quiet rooms, but they weren't always on the ward, sometimes they were off the ward. My own outlet at Napsbury, my quiet room, was the gardens.

There is a sort of hierarchy of wards at Napsbury and other hospitals where some are more acceptable than others. If you were in a hospital which had a unit for people with alcohol problems, in a way they were at the top of the tree. Always there's been a theory that somehow people with alcohol problems, they aren't really mentally ill. They're sort of different, they're kind of superior. We're the ones with mental illness, they don't have mental illness. So, the special unit that would be run on therapeutic community type lines was for people with alcohol problems. Then there is the acute ward – there's a big kind of difference between an acute ward and a long stay ward. I mean, there's not a lot of interaction between the long stay wards and the acute wards – you didn't see a great deal of the people on the long stay wards, you kind of kept with the acute crowd, and the acute ward crowd was obviously superior to the long stay ward because the acute ward was going to go back to the real world in a certain period.

At Napsbury, there was a separate OT for the acute ward people from the one for the long stay ward people, so that was part of the hierarchy. And one of the things that was kind of awful was if you were demoted from an acute ward to a long stay ward. That was a terrible kind of failure, if you like. I remember once, somebody who was actually promoted from a long stay ward to an acute ward, and I remember him kind of appearing and people were not sure how to handle him because in a way he seemed to be a different type of person from us. Then, of course, the other thing was the locked wards or the intensive care unit. It was a possibility that if you were too challenging for the acute ward, you would end up in the locked ward and, of course, that was also something that was a demotion. But the thing that was in a way the least desirable, from our point of view, was the long stay ward. And all these wards were named after trees or shrubs. Larch, Laurel, Acacia, Cyprus, I can't remember them all. And there was a place called The Pines, which was the patients' café. I've forgotten the name of the locked ward, but yes, that was it, someone's been sent to Damson! And that was like a fate worse than death in a way!

Of course, another ward was the rehab ward and that one was relatively OK – to go from an acute ward to a rehab ward. Of course, it was good to go from an acute ward back to the community but if you went from acute ward to a rehab ward, that was certainly not quite as acceptable but not terrible. It still meant that you were on the way back. But people used to spend quite a long time on acute wards even so, although there was a certain limit to the time you could spend on an acute ward.

An important feature of life at Napsbury was the ward round. Ward rounds are very important but very difficult, I think, for patients. They are not that easy for the professionals involved but they are certainly difficult for patients. They usually take place in a small room and there would be at least one psychiatrist there, prob-ably the consultant, and a varying number of other professionals – nurses, occupa-tional therapist, community psychiatric nurse etc. The thing about ward rounds is they are important because they can move you, on if you like, to the next point, and it is where your progress and what happens next is discussed. You may not have that much contact with a psychiatrist during the course of a week and the ward round is an occasion when you are more than likely to see a psychiatrist. It could be your consultant, so it's a significant event. It's up to the consultant basically who goes to a ward round. I think you can possibly say to the nursing staff 'I really want to go to see the doctor today' and that may help to ensure you do go to the ward round. I think a ward round is like an appointment with any health expert – it's anxiety provoking and quite often the fact that you're being interviewed by a number of people – there may be eight or nine people, and quite often you're not introduced to the people and quite often it will just be the psychiatrist talking to you and the rest of the group quite often will not say anything, but listen and watch, so it's kind of a strange experience in a way, a psychodrama where you're performing with the psychiatrist and everyone else is kind of watching and nodding. At the first hospital I was in, Royal Dundee Liff in 1967, the ward round was something like the traditional visit from the consultant you see in films like 'Carry On, Doctor' etc. We would stand at the foot of our beds and the consultant, junior psychiatrist, and two or three of the nursing staff, would come round and we would be interviewed in front of all the other patients – usually for only a couple of minutes.

The big problem for me now is my hearing, because I've got a hearing impairment. Sometimes you're not invited to sit next to the psychiatrist, quite often you're sitting opposite on the other side of the room, that seems to be the traditional position, so it's down to me to ask whether I want to sit next to the psychiatrist because I can't hear. I think I'm fairly good in dealing with ward rounds, one of the things that I do, and I tell other patients to do, is to write down what you want to say, because people come out of ward rounds and say 'I really wanted to say that' and, of course, the thing is you have to wait another week before you can raise that issue again, so it's something you need to prepare for. I think there is always anxiety about are you going to be seen, and it's a bit different from an ordinary hospital appointment where you know you're going to be seen. In this case you don't know whether, or when you, you're going to be seen, and whether it's at ten o clock or one o clock, so the morning of the ward round is a kind of stressful time.

In some ways, it's quite empty, the week between ward rounds, there's not a lot of interaction going on the ward, and that's been a feature of acute ward care in my experience, right back to the sixties. In some ways, it may have got a bit worse. You don't have that much interaction with staff during the time that you are in the ward, partly because there aren't sufficient staff and partly because there's a lot of agency nurses. But I think there is also this culture about qualified nurses spending a lot of time in the nursing office – I think that's always been a feature, and I think it's probably got worse in the last fifteen years because there's more paperwork to be done – reports need to be written, care plans need to be developed, referrals need to be made – there's a lot more bureaucracy, if you like, and that seems to involve nursing staff being in the nursing office a lot. The other thing is that when nursing staff and nursing assistants are on the ward, they're not interacting with patients, they're interacting with each other – reading newspapers, talking to each other rather than talking to inpatients and that I think, again, is something I remember in Napsbury days. I think one of the things that's changed since Napsbury is there's a greater emphasis on observation. Quite a lot of staff are involved in observing individuals who are supposed to be at risk in some way and that all leads to a limited interaction.

A regular feature of life at Napsbury for me, as a permanent non-smoker, would be sitting in the day room with a lot of other patients doing nothing, perhaps with the television on, in a terrible smoky atmosphere. You could see a blue layer that kind of infested the room from about eleven o clock in the morning! It was incredible! My memory is of hours spent doing nothing in Napsbury. Reading, that's what I did the most. Reading and trying to redevelop my concentration. So, I would start off with newspapers and magazines then I would graduate to books and things. But, basically, a lot of time doing nothing. To begin with, with the effects of the medication, I usually had writing problems, I found it quite difficult to write. Occasionally, not in Napsbury but more recently, I've tried to keep a very basic 'what's happened today', not a proper diary, just a few lines on the main events that happened on a particular day, and looking at the writing, I can see to begin with, on the first few days, the writing is very scrawly, very difficult to read, and that's because of the medication.

A couple of the wards I was in in Napsbury had table tennis or small billiard tables, so that was a form of recreation, but basically not a lot. I do remember in Silver Birch, for example, playing scrabble or card games, with nurses being involved in that. That tended to be on the back shift – the afternoon and evening shift when the nurses weren't quite so busy. Once you could move around, obviously you could get out of that environment which made a difference. There was a funny thing on the ward – sometimes, although there's nothing going on it's difficult to do anything. In some ways, it's difficult to concentrate, and you're always waiting for something to happen: there are people maybe acting in strange ways and you observe what's going on, and you're waiting for somebody to do something stupid or for something to happen and it's kind of, well, I've always found it very difficult to think about my problems and the reason why I'm in the acute ward while I'm actually in it there. It's only when I get back home that I have the peace of mind to think about what this all means. I'm not being encouraged to think about what it all means. On the one hand nothing is happening and on the other hand you don't feel kind of able to fill that space with something of your own. I'm not that sure what that's about but maybe it's something to do with the fact that there are a lot of people simply doing nothing and it kind of takes the impetus from you. And there's also the effect of medication – people spend a lot of time sleeping.

And, also, quite a lot of time eating! Eating is a major event. Your day is split up by the main mealtimes. It's the main form of social activity – everybody's involved in it, although there's never that much conversation going on, but it is at least an occasion when most of the ward are together in one place, doing and sharing something. And I can remember in Napsbury, on Silver Birch ward, the kitchen area was always locked, and we kind of waited for the door to be unlocked for breakfast, and then for lunch and then for supper, and when they brought out a pot of tea at various occasions during the day. So, mealtimes themselves are important and there's no shortage of food. It may be that the quality of the food is not that great, but there's no shortage and a thing I always remember at Napsbury was the way they tried to rush you through mealtimes, so you almost didn't have time to start your second course before they were trying to rush everything away and get the squad out who were doing the washing up. So, it always seemed to be quite a hurried event, to rush you through and get you back in the day room again. The other thing is, quite often you would have nurses standing round the ward watching you – quite often it was the only time you saw some of the nurses. They were suddenly all around, at mealtime, and they would stand and watch. Some of them were involved in dishing out the food, the rest were standing there watching. I think they were kind of sharing the occasion, but they were not, because they were not sitting down at a table eating with you, certainly not at Napsbury with patients, and I think it's rare for the staff to eat with patients. On occasions, you could see staff watching people who were supposed to have eating problems. I've seen that happen, in which case a nurse will usually sit at a table, usually the next-door table, and kind of watch them, which I think is objectionable.

But the main thing is the importance of food, certainly to me. At other times of day, when there was nothing going on, eating was also quite an important feature. Going up to the hospital shop during the course of the day and buying sweets or biscuits. And then there was The Pines which was a sort of patients' café in the grounds, and you could go up there and get very cheap bacon and eggs or sandwiches and things like that, and that was a regular part of my routine. I would go up to The Pines, certainly in the afternoon, sometimes after lunch. I would have lunch and then have something to eat up there. The medication was part of the reason – a lot of medication increases your appetite, but also because it is something to do. At Napsbury there was also a place called the Double D which was a restaurant, well a sort of café, just outside the gates to Napsbury, and it was a sort of greasy spoon café and some of us used to go up there. It wasn't part of the hospital, so you had to pay normal prices. The thing about The Pines was it was subsidised, so you had to pay hardly anything for fried egg or whatever. It was very cheap. At Double D you'd get a proper greasy spoon meal and I remember going up there quite often. So, the day was kind of interspersed with eating! Technically, you had to be able to leave the hospital grounds to visit the Double D. I didn't always observe that – it's only about five yards outside the hospital gate so you can bend the rules a little there. I remember going up to Double D after morning OT which might finish at half past eleven, and lunch wasn't until half past twelve. So, I was eating a lot! The thing I remember also in Silver Birch at Napsbury was people would send out for takeaways in the evening so they would have a Chinese or a pizza or whatever. They'd ring up and it would be delivered to the ward door and people would pay their share and sit there eating in the evenings. For some people it was in addition to hospital food. Food was very important. In Napsbury you would normally have to get permission to brew up a pot of tea and you'd go for a pot of tea and bring it out in the day room.

There were other unusual features of the Napsbury environment like the Farm Factory, for instance, which was a sort of alternative to OT for certain people on the acute ward. In some ways it was again talking about hierarchies. It had a lower status than occupational therapy and it used to be often seen as the destination for people who had been in the acute ward quite a while. It consisted of workshops for people doing carpentry and metalwork and things like that and also people might work in the grounds doing manual physical work as opposed to occupational therapy. I don't know why it was called the Farm Factory but people who had been in Napsbury – most of them would say 'I'm going to work in the Farm Factory'. OT was more enjoyable, in my opinion. It involved soccer, tennis in the summer, quizzes and listening to music, music appreciation, some discussion groups, arts and craft groups, some pottery, so quite a range of activities, mostly indoors but outdoors as well, sometimes you would go on walks in the grounds or outside the grounds. Normally there would be a session of OT in the morning and then again in the afternoon and there was a different OT unit for long stay patients. I enjoyed it, and I think some of the things were useful – I used to do quite a lot of artwork and that was kind of helpful. I think, as the hospital ran down, one of the departments that suffered a lot was OT – the premises got smaller, there weren't so many occupational therapists around and I think there tended to be a situation where some of the long stay patients started to mix with the acute patients and I think that affected the kind of OT we did. It became slightly more basic, if you like, and not so many discussions, more quizzes and things like that. Although I enjoyed OT, I think a lot of the patients couldn't see the point of it. I know every morning there was a kind of process where the nursing staff would try to encourage patients to go to OT and it used to be an ongoing struggle because most people didn't want to go. The nursing staff would pursue them with various degrees of energy but quite often they would give up.

I would do anything to get off the ward. So doing something vaguely enjoyable, and maybe constructive, it definitely seemed to me to be a useful way of passing your time rather than sitting in the ward doing nothing. And the occupational therapists were usually very approachable people, they were willing to talk and have a chat and things like that.

3.09

ADAPTED FROM INTERVIEW WITH PETER ABOUT 'THE EXPERIENCE OF ECT'. (*Testimony* 2005, Interviewer: Peter Barham)

[The stanzas of verse quoted below are all from Peter Campbell's unpublished poem '*Waiting for ECT*']

Waiting for ECT
Is like waiting for a train.
A non-stop Inter City
Flashing through the tunnels
Of your brain.

We trace descent to Frankenstein,
To Wolfman and the Zongoid from the Marsh.
We pinch at chair arms in our unrefined condition,
We are broke down
And someone's called the electricians.
Are there some questions just too rational to ask?

Waiting for ECT
Is like living on the pale
And wondering
Cannot hands and voices heal me?

P1   Can we start by talking about your experience of ECT, and the question of consent?

P2   I suppose I've had three courses of ECT on different occasions during different admissions in the early 1970s, and I can't honestly remember giving my consent at all. I don't remember signing anything, I don't really remember giving consent.

    DOI: 10.4324/9781003636434-44

P1   Not on any occasion?

P2   No, I think it's possible on a couple of occasions I was simply told – 'Well you're going to have ECT' and I said to myself 'OK – that's what they're recommending and I don't think there's much I can do about it'. There was one occasion when they said they were going to give me ECT and I was a voluntary patient, and I said they can't give it because I was voluntary and I remember going to a social worker and complaining, but what happened in the end, they said to me I was voluntary but if I didn't agree to ECT they would section me, so I just acquiesced and was not put on a section, and so that was the kind of situation. I've got a feeling that consent has become much more of an issue than it used to be, particularly maybe since the 1983 Mental Health Act. These occasions were before then. I think the whole issue of consent, the whole formality, is probably different. I've got no personal experience of that, but I think it may be less likely that people are given ECT without going through the consent process – that's my feeling about ECT itself.

P1   Before we go to the experience itself, you don't recall having any conversations with doctors where the issue of ECT was discussed, it was just presented to you as something that had been decided for you, kind of thing.

P2   To be honest, I can't remember having a full discussion at any point. I can't be categorical about that, but I certainly don't think that ECT was ever explained to me, what the procedure was. Maybe they said something about the possible negative effects, like headache, and maybe disorientation, and perhaps a bit of memory loss around the period of the actual treatment. I don't remember ever being given a kind of explanation of what was going to happen. I think I just found that out from going through it, so I certainly wasn't given any written explanation. I think it's possible that it was kind of explained to me, the general reasons why they were going to give me ECT, but that was about all.

P1   Do you remember discussing it with other patients at the time? Do you have a sense of what the kind of common perception of ECT was within the patients' subculture?

P2   ECT is feared, and it's looked upon in a negative way. I remember the first time I was ever in hospital in Dundee, I was eighteen or something like that. I remember, within a week or so of being in the hospital, of being aware that ECT was a possibility, and it was something you didn't want to happen. It was a kind of last resort thing you might have. The fact that it was kind of feared, and looked at negatively, and the fact that it was a kind of last resort to have, kind of at the end of the line if other things didn't work.

P1   I mean, this was the era of '*One Flew Over the Cuckoo's Nest*' after all.

P2   That's right. I remember a patient in the ward who had had ECT saying 'Oh this could be what you'll be given' and I think he was trying to scare me a bit. At that point, the chances of me being given ECT were pretty low, but it was definitely on the menu and the fact that it was kind of feared, and looked at negatively, and the fact that it was kind of a last resort, and the feeling that if

181

you do have to have ECT that shows your problems are really serious, I suppose you could say there is a sort of stigma around ECT, and people who had to have ECT were at the bottom of the pile.

P1 The intractables, yes.

P2 Yes, the intractables, that's right. So, I think within the patient culture ECT is something you want to avoid almost at all costs, and I knew on two or three occasions patients who were very upset. I remember on one occasion, when I was in Epsom District Hospital, there was a particular woman who was on a course of ECT and she got very agitated, and was crying almost inconsolably, on every evening before the following morning when she was to be given ECT, and she would get very upset. In West Park, I remember on occasions when I was waiting for ECT, there was a woman who was brought from another ward and she also got extremely agitated, and I remember her coming, and she was so distressed, you could kind of hear her coming up the stairs to the treatment room, and they would take her into the treatment room almost always immediately – she didn't wait around for it.

Obviously ECT is a controversial treatment. I think it is controversial in terms of the mental health field and I think among service users and survivors it is kind of more controversial and I think their opposition is even greater. It's a bit like a kind of monster looming in the background. When I was in hospital quite recently – the year before last-there was a possibility that I might be given ECT as I was in a sort of catatonic state. They told me afterwards that if I hadn't pulled out of it, they were afraid it might be life threatening, or it might be quite damaging to me physically, so the possibility was of giving me ECT. I was actually quite opposed to that, and I have written an advance directive saying that I don't want to be given ECT unless it's the very last resort. Of course, I know that it's an advance directive, but when it comes down to it, it is the psychiatrist's decision, and if the psychiatrist thinks it's life-threatening, they will give me ECT without my consent. Probably, when I was in this kind of catatonic state, I wouldn't be able, or be fully aware, of what was going on anyway. So, I think ECT is something that people fear, they're opposed to. It's kind of there in the background, it's a possibility, particularly if you are depressed, that's something that might happen at the end of the line.

P1 But for you personally, going through it, actually being subjected to ECT, did you feel, in some sense, that it was a kind of radicalising experience for you? A formative experience in your feeling about psychiatry, and about yourself in the mental health system? I mean, by comparison with seclusion and other focal experiences?

P2 Yes, I think it was. I think I kind of felt it was a mistreatment. I questioned whether it was necessary. It didn't feel good. The actual process made me feel in some way, inhuman. I think psychologically it is quite damaging – ECT, because in a way it seems like a mechanical treatment, and it's not very pleasant and I don't think you're given a lot of support about this. Certainly, in the days when I had it, you weren't. It is something about, how have I really got into this position, where talking and support no longer work, and I've got to be given this kind of unpleasant mechanical intervention? And certainly, being given it against my will, I certainly think that that radicalised me. I think being given any treatment against your will radicalises you, but I think that situation I explained to you earlier about being a voluntary patient when I refused ECT, and they were basically saying 'well we will put you on a section and you will have to have it then', that seems to me unacceptable, and it kind of shows just how powerless you are.

P1   It's a classic double bind.

P2   That's right, exactly. I mean the other thing I remember very clearly was the first time I was given a course of ECT in Banstead hospital – that was possibly 1971. How they did it in those days, it was a kind of Nightingale ward, and people who were going to have ECT were all lying on beds in the ward, and basically they came up the row doing ECT with the machine, so you could kind of hear it going on for each of the people, and they gradually worked their way up towards you, and I've got this vivid picture of my being kind of towards the end of the ward, so it was quite a long process of them going through treating people and moving up, there were eight or nine people, because I think in those days it was used much more than it is now. I think it would be quite uncommon to have eight or nine people at one session nowadays.

P1   So was there no privacy there? Did they not put screens around?

P2   There were screens but nothing else. I think it was the fact that you could kind of hear what was going on – the doctors and the nurses, kind of muttering, and then the beds being moved after the ECT had been done, the beds were pushed to the other side of the ward, where people could recover. And just kind of waiting there, as they move closer to you, and I remember one of the things was, because I am so tall, I was very worried about the fact that my legs, well the back of my ankles, were resting on the metal bar at the bottom of the bed, and I remember worrying that if they gave me electric shock with my ankles resting on the metal, what would happen with the electricity? Just a crazy thought, but I remember that. So, I think that is always something I wouldn't forget, and that emphasises my feeling that it was an undignified kind of treatment and insensitively administered. And I remember other times I had ECT, it was done in the ECT suite, and so you went in, and you waited your turn in a waiting room, and you went through, and you were given it on your own, and then you were wheeled into another room to recover. Another thing I remember, was that because I was pretty controlled, pretty self-possessed, I used to be taken to the waiting room quite early, I would be sitting in the waiting room, and because I was quite self-possessed and seemed to be handling the waiting OK, I would quite often have to wait a long time and people who arrived later would be taken first, so I used to have to sit there for quite long periods and I remember walking across – this was in West

Park – I remember walking right from one side of the hospital to the other, this was under escort, to have ECT and I mean the treatment itself had kind of negative effects. They wouldn't be that extreme with me. I remember having slight headaches immediately afterwards when I came to, a bit disoriented, but in terms of long-term memory loss, I don't think it has had any effect on me, in terms of my learning ability or things like that – that seems to be OK. Whether it did any good, that's difficult to say. I mean, I was given ECT and I got better eventually, but I was also given a load of other things – when I was given ECT, I was on a major tranquilliser, possibly even a minor tranquilliser as well, so God knows what worked.

P1   So there was no particular sense of it shaking you out of one state into something else?

P2   Not really. I think probably there was an occasion when I was quite depressed, then the depression finished and I got onto a better level and I suppose it is possible that on that occasion the ECT did help me move on from my depression, but I think in those days ECT wasn't a last resort to the extent that it seems to be now. When I was in Banstead, I was only in Banstead for a short while before they gave me ECT – it was only a couple of weeks, so it wasn't really a last resort. I mean I can't remember whether I was put on antidepressants before I was given ECT but the fact that I was given it so quickly suggests that they didn't give the antidepressants, if I was given them, very much time. But I think that in the early 1970s, ECT was much more common, there's no doubt about that, and I think that the figures probably reflect that as well, that ECT was more likely if you were depressed and fairly deeply depressed, it was quite likely you were given ECT. And I remember three or four people being quite regularly on ECT during the time I was in hospital.

P1   How many treatments were there in a course of ECT – remind me?

P2   Somewhere around six – I think it's usually six or eight. I always say that I probably had around eighteen ECTs, three courses of six. I can't remember exactly.

P1   And they were on consecutive days?

P2   No twice a week – it's usually twice a week, Monday and Thursday, that sort of thing, usually a couple of days in between. I'm not sure, maybe people were given less, but I think, when you talked about ECT, it's normally about six. And then they would wait for maybe a couple of weeks or so, I think, before they would start another course. But I've met people, I've seen people who it seems to have benefited, and I have certainly spoken to people and read about people who say ECT has helped them – they would willingly undergo the treatment again. I think there is this dreadful thing about depression – anything that can move you through it, it seems very desirable – and I've known one or two people who are quite critical about psychiatry, and critical about physical treatment as a whole, but when they have been depressed they have actually thought well, maybe ECT would help me, and I think you've got to recognise maybe ECT can be helpful.

P1 Mmmm

P2 And I wouldn't, for example, want to ban ECT. I think there is a section of the survivor movement who would like to ban ECT. I think it is a treatment that can work and it can also damage people – I think there is evidence that it can also damage people long term, in terms of memory loss and things like that, but I think if it can help, if there is a possibility of it helping, and people are given the information about the pros and cons and the alternatives, and they make a free choice – as far as you can ever make a free choice if you are an inpatient in a psychiatric unit – and people are saying – 'yes do this' – in some ways, even if you are a voluntary patient, it is very difficult to say 'no I won't do this'. But if people are given the opportunity to consent, and they are given the full information and there are other alternatives available, then I think ECT is a legitimate possibility and I wouldn't want to deny that to people, particularly, as I say, as there are a substantial number of people who say ECT was helpful in the past and they willingly, you know, undertake it again. The other problem is, you hear of people who have had hundreds of ECTs, and that must raise questions to me about how effective it is. I mean, maybe it's effective in the short term, maybe it does accelerate peoples' recovery but I kind of think of, how come these people are having so many ECTs, and also one of the things you sometimes hear about is psychiatrists apparently saying, 'we'll just bring you in and top you up with ECT'.

P1 I have not heard that expression before.

P2 Yes, I've heard it, I've definitely heard it. I can't remember how I came across it but I've definitely heard it – 'Oh we'll just top you up with a few ECT's' which I think is a revealing phrase. And I think ECT can be abused, and I think again that is less likely nowadays because it's not used so much, and there are certain psychiatrists who never, or almost never, use ECT. I think the unit that I now use – I can't remember anybody being given ECT. In fact, I don't think they do it at Edgware. If they really decide you need ECT, you have to go to another hospital for it – I think Chase Farm, which is in the same trust but is a different hospital.

I actually think there is something – this may sound kind of contradictory, but I think there is something inherently demeaning about the treatment, even if it is beneficial. I think there is something about having electric currents pass through your brain and I think it is something to do with this sort of Frankenstein feeling about it.

That's how it feels. I mean I think personally that I would avoid ECT at all costs, almost all costs – if it saved my life, maybe not, but anything short of that, I would try to avoid ECT.

P1 I understand that. Would you advise somebody else to do the same? Is that the advice you would give?

P2 No, I mean I don't think I would say – 'Whatever you do, don't have ECT'. I think I would point out the negative aspects, and I think I would argue for them considering the alternatives very seriously and for them having, I mean, basically people have got to make their mind up for themselves.

185

P1   Right.

P2   I think I would say, 'Well I've found it a demeaning treatment. I am not con-vinced it worked for me,' but I would also say I know people who don't feel that way at all. But, I mean, I think there are risks attached to ECT, and I think people need to be aware of them.

    I think I've probably always felt damaged psychologically by the way ECT was used on me. I think I probably felt that less strongly at the time I was in hospital but after that, on reflection, I probably felt more strongly, and more angry about it. I think being in the company of people who feel similarly in the survivor movement, because there are very few people in the survivor movement who are actually in favour of ECT, and would actively like to see ECT used more, and be more available, so it is part of the culture, so I think that kind of heightened my feeling. But probably, before I was ever involved in the survivor movement, probably the first poem I ever wrote, about the psychiatric system, and certainly the first poem I ever performed, or ever came out with in public, was a poem about ECT. Waiting for ECT is like wait-ing for a train. A non-stop inter-city flashing through the panels of your brain, and then it goes on to talk about Frankenstein, I can't remember the words off hand but that was certainly the first poem I ever wrote about psychiatry and that was going back to that image in West Park, waiting in the waiting room to have ECT and that woman who is very upset – hearing her coming up the stairs. I think I have always felt very strongly about ECT before I got involved in the survivor movement.

    One of the things is that ECT doesn't feel like a caring intervention. I think there are ways you can perhaps make it a more caring intervention, and perhaps now it is handled more sensitively than it used to be, but I'm not sure about that. I certainly think the way I have experienced it, personally, it wasn't a very caring package.

Ourselves are not unchanged.
We did not ask for this.
A casual hand, one tea,
Our name in red upon the escort's list.
This does not meet our questions or our needs
A course of seven treatments and godspeed'

That's how it feels.
We touch the cold untruth.
We do not need the textbooks or the proof.
We speak as Man,
We would be spoken to.
Our souls are not machines
That need be broken into.

3.10

ADAPTED FROM INTERVIEW WITH PETER ABOUT 'THE EXPERIENCE OF PSYCHOTROPIC DRUGS'. (*Testimony* 2005, Interviewer: Peter Barham)

P2 In the early days I think, and for quite a while, I was pretty unquestioning in many respects. When it comes down to it, for the last 37 years I have been on medication for most of that time, so in terms of my opposition to medication, I have actually been taking medication for most of the time. I think in that first asylum, the thing I remember is Chloral Hydrate, which is a medication used since the middle of the nineteenth century, and I think in the late 1960s it was still being used quite widely, and the way it was used on me was they were knock out drops you could get if you couldn't get to sleep.

P1 The liquid cosh.

P2 Yes, the liquid cosh. I don't remember if I was on sleeping tablets at night, but I had the medication at night, and then you had to judge it. If you couldn't get to sleep, you had to judge it just right when you got up and said to the nurses at the office that you can't sleep. If you got up too early, they would send you back to try and get to sleep. If you got up too late, they wouldn't give you Chloral Hydrate because you'd be stupefied the following morning. So, you had to judge it just right and they would give you Chloral Hydrate and that would knock you out. Certainly, in the early stages of my admission, when I was very anxious and sleep was very difficult, I think the knowledge that there was something that would knock you out in some ways was helpful.

That was my first encounter with medication. And when I was discharged, I was on medication, Chlorpromazine, for a period of years, and taking it regularly, not suffering too many negative effects, certainly no noticeable

DOI: 10.4324/9781003636434-45

negative effects. Certainly, dry mouth that was a problem, but other negative effects I didn't really experience.

P1   In terms of your creative processes as it were?

P2   Oh yes, my creative processes it did affect, yes, and there was a period when I was on depot injections. I think that whole period from, say, 1967 and the following ten years, I think my creativity was affected, and it wasn't really until I was put on lithium for a period of years that I think my creativity came back and that was a period when I started writing poetry again. I used to write poetry as an adolescent and then there was this period for about ten years when my creativity really was affected. I would abhor to be put back on depot injections. There was a time in the early 1990s when it was suggested that maybe I should go back on depot injections, and I was devastated. It's almost the same as my feelings about ECT – depot injections are just like the curtains coming down.

P1   They make you very drowsy.

P2   They make you drowsy, and your perception and kind of appreciation of what's going on in the world, your concentration…

P1   A dumbing down experience?

P2   Just being dumbed down, being held down. In some ways I was doing ok on depot injections. I wasn't having so many crises, but the quality of my life was circumscribed, it was diminished basically. So, as I say, I would sooner not be on depot injections and have crises every so often, than be on depot injections and not have crises. I wouldn't want to ever go back on depot injections, ever, ever. I think I've been on medication far too much. Looking back, I don't think it was necessary for me to be on Chlorpromazine, or depot injections, all the time. I think one of my feelings about medication is that I think medication can be very helpful in a crisis. I am much less sure about how useful medication is taking it all the time, although I think there is this contradiction, as I have been taking medication all the time. I always find it very difficult to take the plunge and say I'm not going to take medication at all. There's been a couple of occasions when I've almost got there, not in opposition to the psychiatrist, but working with the psychiatrist, but then something has gone wrong and, of course, the argument then is that if you'd stayed on the medication you wouldn't have a crisis and that kind of argument and the argument of, well, 'you're doing ok on your medication why come off it', are very strong arguments. The psychiatrist may say you're taking a big risk, you're ok on your medication. One psychiatrist said to me, if you stop taking your medication you'll be readmitted within a month, so it is quite difficult to go against the expert and take that kind of plunge on my own responsibility. I mean, I've got a number of friends who have done that and have done it reasonably successfully. I've got some friends who've done it and live quite a distressing life, or certainly a life which has periods of distress in it, which they chose to go through rather than take medication. Even though I kind of see that people can survive, and survive quite well without medication, I haven't been able to do that myself.

P1 You seem to almost imply that's a kind of weakness. But, to be the devil's advocate, one could argue the opposite, that actually you function very well, you obviously – you and lithium seem to do rather well together, you lead a creative life....

P2 I think what is an interesting issue is, why do we feel it is a weakness to be on psychiatric drugs?

P1 It's my word but that's what you imply – is that right?

P2 I think I feel it is a weakness, and I think a large number of people with a mental illness diagnosis feel it's a weakness to be on medication. I am not really sure that I know a convincing answer to that, but I think there is a sort of thing about – going back to this kind of thing about pull yourself together, or be a real adult – some kind of feeling that we should, and we want to, sort these problems out ourselves, and that is something to do with self-worth, I suppose, self-esteem, and for some reason medication seems to be seen as a weakness. And maybe it's tied up with this whole idea of admitting that your problems are a medical issue – for some people, anyway, they don't believe it, they don't feel that's what it is about. I think there is no doubt that I do feel that it's a weakness to use psychiatric drugs, although that isn't logical and it's a feeling.

P1 It's obviously tied up with psychiatric power in some way – the power of the doctor and the idea that it is somehow an imposition, which it often is, of course, but you could argue that in your case, at this point in time, it's now freely chosen by yourself, that you have other options, but nevertheless on consideration you have chosen this option – to stick with the lithium.

P2 Yes, I think I have chosen and accept the need to use psychiatric drugs and I think the issue for me, for a period of years, has been about minimising the number of drugs that I'm on, minimising my use of drugs, because I think there is no doubt that these drugs do damage, or can damage you physically, and if I look back I think almost all, if not all, of the medications that I have been on long term, if you like maintenance type medications – almost all of them have ended up damaging me physically. Lithium affected my thyroid, carbamazepine gave me agranulocytosis which is a blood disorder. The drug that I am currently on seems to have affected my platelet blood count, though not seriously enough to justify coming off the drug or making it necessary to come off the drug. I think there's no doubt that, in my experience these drugs have damaged me physically or the long-term use of them has damaged me physically, and I think there is a good reason for me to want to be on as few medications as possible, and at one time I was on just a maintenance dose of antidepressants and an anti-psychotic, and now I'm just on a maintenance dose of an anti-psychotic and I have been in great argument with my psychiatrist about whether or not I need an anti-psychotic and that's a kind of unresolved argument. I am taking an anti-psychotic at the moment, on a very low dose, but my aim would be to come off that, but I think there is no doubt that drugs have been an issue of contention, a major issue of contention between me and the psychiatrist, throughout my career in the system. It has quite often been an issue to do with dosages, rather than coming off medication altogether, and whether it's necessary to be on more than one medication, and all those sorts of things. Partly it's to do with power – struggling against the power of the psychiatrist, and the way of doing that is to argue about medication because obviously that's one of the big areas of the psychiatrist's power – they may be experts on medication and they say if you don't take your medication, awful things will happen.

P1   You implied somehow, there's also been a shift in your experience – this is what I pick up, your experience now with the psychiatrist is less adversarial than it was, more a creative, open-ended exchange.

P2   Yes, I think that in recent years there's been more of a discussion possible, whereas I think going back, perhaps it was more adversarial and perhaps I was taking a more extreme position, whereas in recent years I was saying I want to reduce medication and I've found psychiatrists who are prepared to reduce medication over a period of time, so you're on as little medication as possible, and I think that maybe I've come to accept that as being the most possible goal. I think that one of the important things is, I've got much more information about medication than I used to have in the 1970s and 1980s. I know more about medication than I used to, and I have been given more information than I used to, and on one occasion, when I was being changed from one drug to another, my community psychiatric nurse (CPN) – the mental health equivalent of a district nurse operating 'in the community' – photocopied a whole lot of information from the drugs textbook and gave it to me. There's also been things like the Maudsley phone-in line where you can phone in and talk to a pharmacist about medications. So, I am in a much better situation to discuss what's going on. Finally, after years and years, it got through to psychiatrists that despite the fact that I would argue about medication, I was not a notorious non-complier and in fact, if I said I will take my medication, I would always take it.

When I stopped taking my medication it would be because I'm in a crisis. I'd be so confused that I stopped taking my medication. There have been occasions when I was in a crisis and I can't actually remember whether I have taken my medication or not, so I've not taken it, and maybe I should've taken it. For many years I was always accused of stopping taking my medication and ending up in a crisis. But it is not to do with that – it's to do with being in a crisis and stopping taking my medication. I think the other thing about my feelings on medication is that, apart from depot injections, I don't think there's any medication that's going to stop me having a crisis. If the conditions are so severe, I'm going to have a crisis whether I'm on medication or not. I mean, not taking my medication because I'm in a crisis may make that crisis more severe.

The other thing I find very interesting, and I feel extremely frustrated about, is the fact I am not allowed to have access to sleeping pills. That's a no and has been for quite a number of years. I used to use sleeping pills in the hospital back in the 1970s, but in the last fifteen years or so it's been impossible for me to get a prescription for a sleeping pill through psychiatrists.

P1   Why?

P2   Good question. I think because they're addictive, the possibility of their being addictive. I think there is also the fact that some of the major tranquillisers in use now are supposed to help you sleep, so rather than give me a sleeping tablet, they'll say take this anti-psychotic and that'll help you sleep. But my argument has been quite often that what I need is sleep – when I'm in a crisis, I stop sleeping, and what I need is sleep, and if I had a few sleeping tablets I would sleep, and that would prevent me from spiralling into a deep crisis.

P1   Sleeping tablets are addictive but you actually have to take them for quite some time, for them to become addictive, so the kind of usage you're talking about, take them for a week to help you through a crisis, you're not going to be an addict after that!

P2   Maybe overdose is another thing they're concerned about, but it has just been a blank wall. They might say, well, you might get so confused, you might take them unintentionally, so to speak. But that's the way it is, and it's an issue which doesn't seem to be open to negotiation, certainly not with the regime I'm living under at the moment. It doesn't seem to be justifiable really. I would have thought, if we are trying out all these ways of preventing me having a crisis, diminishing the severity of the crisis, which has been a development over the last fifteen years. I have been working quite hard over the years, in partnership with the CPN, and with the psychiatrist, to address this issue of my crises, to address the issue of my crisis in all possible ways, but to address the issue with sleeping tablets is not possible. It seems to me it is sensible to say, 'let's try it – see if it works'. But that's the power of the psychiatrist and, of course, the psychiatrist has decided that, basically, I have a psychotic element in my make-up and I should take an anti-psychotic all the time. I am willing to admit that, when I have a crisis, that crisis has signs of psychotic behaviour and thought, but I don't think that necessarily means I should take anti-psychotics all the time, particularly as they act very quickly. So if I was to take anti-psychotics over the period when I was in a crisis, or likely to be in a crisis situation, that's how I would rather do it – self-management, if you like, rather than taking these things in a blanket way.

P1   So those are the two fronts where you encounter resistance – on the anti-psychotic issue and on the sleeplessness question.

P2   Yes, I think in other ways some of my concern about medication has been met, in terms of information, in terms of monitoring, so I think that has changed quite a lot from the ways things were. I remember when I was on depot injections, in the 1970s, I wasn't given information about the negative effects of depot injections. I used to get what is called oculogyric crises which is basically a fixation of the eyeball, so a few days after a depot I used to find my vision got fixated on the horizon or if I was in a room, I would find

191

I was staring at the ceiling and couldn't stop myself. Then I would basically go home and go to bed and when I woke up it seemed to have gone away. I had no idea this was connected to depot injections. I had no idea that it was connected with depot injections. I did nothing about it and then one day my knees seized up, I couldn't walk. I was going somewhere and I had to go home and drag myself the last 100 yards, dragging myself along the pavement. I went to the hospital the next day and they said it was a side effect of the injection I was on and gave me an intramuscular injection of Kemadrin. And so from then on I was taking Kemadrin alongside my injection, but they never told me that. When I was returned to the community, they never gave me that information, and when I was put on lithium originally, I was told 'Oh Lithium is not like psychotropic drugs, it doesn't have such negative effects'. Well, that is bullshit! I mean, lithium has a load of negative effects as I found out myself, and you've got to monitor lithium, you've got to have blood tests, because the difference between a therapeutic and a toxic level is very small. I was given the impression that lithium is fine, you don't have to worry about lithium, it doesn't have negative effects, it's a salt, it doesn't have negative effects, it's not like a manufactured drug. And again, we're talking about a long time ago – the 1970s- and I think there has been a significant shift about the amount of information that people are given. Whether people are given full information, I think is a different matter and I think that if you look at the surveys, large numbers of psychiatric drug users would say, 'I don't think we get enough information'. I think something like 70 per cent of people would say that. I certainly think people get more information than they used to, and I certainly think it is easier to find information from other places than your CPN or your psychiatrist.

3.11

'THE SURVIVOR MOVEMENT IN THE 1980s' (2006)

I'm really delighted to be here today and would like to thank Colin Gell and the other organisers for inviting me. I've been moving flat for the last couple of weeks and I've been totally focused on moving. I've been trying to move for the last three years and I've finally made it, so this is my first excursion back into the outside world again. It's nice to get out of my flat, it's nice to get out of London, it's nice to come up to Birmingham. It's also good to contribute to an event that is celebrating service user action, service user involvement, whatever you want to call it. It used to be called self-advocacy in the 1980s, we used to talk about self-advocacy but that seems to be a phrase of the past. Anyway, it's good to be able to talk about and celebrate service user action, because I think there are things worth celebrating, and I think it's useful to be aware of and look at our history and that informs us about how maybe we can do things better in the future.

So I'm going to talk about things that have happened over the last 20 years that I think are interesting and important. I'm not going to try to provide a balanced history. What I am talking about are my personal impressions, and I'm going to focus on things that I know most about. The period 1985 to 1995 was when I was most involved at a national level, so I will focus quite a bit on that decade. I want to say a little bit about what my own involvement has been so you get an idea of what my perspective is. I got involved in things in the 1980s really, the early 1980s. I'd moved to a new part of London, I'd been unemployed or under-employed for a number of years, and I decided to give up trying to have a conventional career and decided that I would try to change things in the mental health field, and I thought the only way of doing that was to get involved in MIND. I wasn't aware at that point of any service user organisations, I was only aware of MIND. So I got involved in

Adapted from two versions on file of Peter's opening address at the "TWO DECADES OF CHANGE: CELEBRATING USER INVOLVEMENT" day conference in Birmingham on 2 November 2006. An accessible pdf of the proceedings edited by Marion Clark and Tony Glynn is on Andrew Robert's website at: http://studymore.org.uk/twodec.pdf

DOI: 10.4324/9781003636434-46

MIND in Camden, which is a local MIND organisation, as a volunteer. Through them I got involved in setting up a local service user group which was called Camden Mental Health Consortium, which was one of the first local action groups in London and still exists. It's been going since 1986, so it's a long running group. At the same time as I was involved in Camden Mental Health Consortium, I made contact with two other groups which were more radical, more campaigning groups, one of which was called The Campaign Against Psychiatric Oppression (CAPO) and the other one was called British Network for Alternatives to Psychiatry.

CAPO was a service user/survivor only group, quite a small radical, separatist network group. British Network for Alternatives to Psychiatry was largely London-based and it was made up of mental health workers and service users. It was through my involvement with MIND in Camden that I got invited to get a bit involved with National MIND and I went to the 1985 MIND Annual Conference, in Kensington. There was a meeting of service users immediately afterwards and from that meeting Survivors Speak Out was founded and I was involved as an officer in Survivors Speak Out from 1986 to 1996, so that was my main national involvement during that period. Then in 1991, I was involved in setting up Survivors Poetry, with three other survivor poets and for two or three years I was very involved with that, and I am still involved with Survivors Poetry, but not to such a great degree. From the early 1990s I became a freelance trainer, earning my living by doing teaching work mainly, and so that's been being involved in the education field, which has been my main area of activity for the past fifteen years or so.

So that's my own personal story of being involved. It seems to me that it's important to celebrate service user/survivor action, and that seems to me to be a key feature of what we should be doing today. And I wanted to start off by saying what it has meant to me personally, not so much what it's done to change the world, if it has done anything, but what it's actually done in terms of having an influence on my life, and it certainly changed my life totally for the better.

In the early 1980s and before the 1980s, basically I was adrift. I'd gone into mental health services for the first time in 1967 and for the next fifteen years I was going in and out of hospital, adrift, beneath the surface as much as on top of the surface, isolated, alienated from myself, from other people, carrying a whole lot of negative baggage around with me about who I was, what my problems were, that I was suffering from a mental illness all these kind of things. Silenced. I had no voice at all. Meeting other survivors who wanted to change things, who felt the same thing about their life, and who wanted to change things, totally transformed my life. It changed the way I thought about my own experiences and the experiences of other people. I realised that other people felt the same way as I did about how mental health services had treated them. Other people had the same kind of interior experiences as I did, paranoia, psychotic episodes and whatever, and that made a great deal of difference to me. I have also learned a lot about other difficulties that I don't have. For example, hearing voices, self-harm, areas that I was frightened about or had been repelled by, and through meeting survivors with those experiences I have learned a tremendous amount about whole areas of mental distress which I never knew about before.

Meeting other survivors has helped me cope better with my own distress. I've had tremendous good fortune in having a number of close survivor friends who have helped me through a series of distressing episodes. One of the most memorable things that's happened to me is actually having a survivor who is a friend of mine, be my advocate. I'll never forget when I first had an advocate accompanying me into a ward round, and having a survivor acting as my advocate there made a tremendous difference. Having people who would simply accept, 'OK, here you are, occasionally you do lose it, you lose control, you become very strange, you do things you wouldn't normally do, but that's OK, we all have phases like that'. Being accepted with the difficulties I have by other survivors has made a tremendous difference to my life.

My own self-esteem was transformed. In a way I have been liberated. I was able to take all those negative experiences in my life that I had to hide, I couldn't talk to anybody about, that I was ashamed of, and share them with other people. I was able to think about them, analyse them and use them in a constructive way. People listened to me and us collectively, and actually learnt from us and respected and valued our views. That has made an enormous change to the way I think about myself, to my whole life in general and to my feeling that I had a worthwhile life. I've done a lot of interesting things. I've been able to travel around the country, meeting other service users, talk at conferences, teach here and there. I've been able to develop teaching skills. I've been able to do creative writing, to write poetry, to write prose, to have articles published, to learn skills, and all those things would probably have never happened in my life, if I hadn't actually had the good fortune to meet up with other service users and survivors and get involved in service user/survivor action.

All of this hasn't made a tremendous difference to my life in terms of stopping me going into mental hospitals. I continue to do that regularly, but in every other way, it's transformed my life completely. I dislike people talking about service action as being therapeutic, that to me is not what service user action is about. But I have to say that it certainly has changed my life for the better, and I think we shouldn't overlook the transformation that being involved in action can have on individuals, regardless of whether we are actually changing anything.

Whether we've achieved anything, whether we've got anything to celebrate in terms of what we've achieved in the real world, is a more controversial matter. But I think looking back at our history, the important thing to remember when we are trying to work out what changes have happened is that before the early 1980s, service users were not involved. We were not involved in our own care and treatment. There were no patients' councils, no advocacy and very little information. I think it's worth remembering that now we talk about advocacy as being essential. We argue about the need to have a right to advocacy for people who are detained under the Mental Health Act. Indeed, a right to advocacy for service users as a whole. But in the early 1980s advocacy was never talked about. There wasn't any. It wasn't on the menu at all. So we weren't properly involved in our own care and treatment because there was no advocacy. We were not involved in the development of services in any meaningful way either. We were not involved in consultation. We were not involved in training. We were not involved in research. We were not involved in providing our own services. We simply weren't involved.

If you look at the 1983 Mental Health Act, that was developed without any significant input from service users. And if you look at what is happening at the moment, when we've been arguing for years about amending the Mental Health Act, service users have certainly had the opportunity to be involved in this process and make a contribution. Whatever our influence has been is a different matter but certainly we've been there, we've had the opportunity to speak out about the Mental Health Act, and that certainly didn't happen when the 1983 Mental Health Act was being developed.

We were not involved in debates about understandings about what madness, distress, mental illness is. Nobody listened to us. Nobody thought we had anything worthwhile to say about our own experiences because we were mentally ill, we couldn't possibly have any 'insight' into what our lives were about. That has changed. We were not meaningfully involved in major voluntary organisations. National MIND in the early 1980s saw themselves as being the 'voice of the mentally ill'. But they didn't consult us, they had no mechanisms to make themselves sensitive to what service users really thought. Rethink, or the National Schizophrenia Fellowship, as it was then, was an organisation which basically represented the views of relatives. At that time all the major voluntary mental health organisations were not in tune with service users, service users were not meaningfully involved, they had no power or influence over these organisations. At the same time there were no service user organisations and service user controlled or service user only organisations. No independent organisations except very few.

Basically we were nowhere. Silent, excluded, outside the room rather than inside the room, that was it. And I think it's important now that service user involvement is established and accepted and seen as being a good thing, just to remember that 20 years ago – there wasn't any. I think the other thing worth being aware of is we had to fight for it. This wasn't something that the service providers or the government suddenly woke up to and said, 'oh yeah this is a good idea, let's do it'. This was something that we had to fight for and struggle for. It was not of course just service users and service user activists who brought about this change. There were also people running the mental health system who thought it was a good idea. But service user involvement was not something that everybody thought was a good idea, far from it. It was not something that was granted to us, we had to fight for it.

During the early years, certainly most of the 1980s and the early 1990s, we were having to make the case for 'Why involve service users?' So almost every time I remember going to any event, the first five minutes at least of anything I ever said, was basically establishing the case for 'Why listen to service users?' 'What are the reasons for doing that?' and we had to go through that time and time again. Why it was a good idea to involve service users? There was a great deal of opposition to this. The basic position most people took was sceptical. Most mental health

196

workers certainly took a sceptical position. There was a great deal of obstruction. There were a number of techniques to obstruct what we were trying to do. One of them was the question of 'Who is a service user?' I don't know whether you have ever come up against that argument. But what used to happen was that you'd go to a meeting about service involvement. I remember going to one at the Institute of Psychiatry, where the entire morning was taken up with a debate by eminent psychiatrists about who a service user was. They decided that they couldn't do anything about involving service users, until they decided who a service user was.

To me it has always seemed obvious who a service user is. To me this debate was a clear obstruction technique. 'We can't do anything until we decide who we're talking about'. Representativeness was another one. 'Oh you're not representative, we can't listen to you because you're not a typical service user', all that kind of thing, and that's one that continues to this day. One of the things I remember, there was tremendous anger from many mental health workers about the idea that we wanted to set up our own groups, that we didn't want mental health workers in our groups, we wanted service user only groups. I remember going to one conference in York. I remember the workshop I was in had to be abandoned because the mental health workers in it were so angry that we didn't want them to be involved in our groups. So there was a tremendous lot of scepticism, opposition, obstruction, anger. I mean there was a lot of 'Who are these people? Who are these people coming out of the woodwork and telling us you've done nasty things to us, why have you done this?' Being angry, being emotional, but not only being angry and emotional but actually having good arguments as well. And that's what's hard to take. If someone is angry and emotional you can dismiss them, but if they've actually got good arguments then it's more difficult. So there was a good deal of hostility and resentment.

I remember going to the Common Concerns Conference in 1998, a big conference in Brighton, with service users from other countries, and it was about half service users and half mental health workers. It was an extremely confrontational conference. For one thing service users took over the agenda, we changed the whole agenda at the beginning of the conference and said we don't want it done that way. But there was also a lot of hostility and most of the workshops were being run by service users. I remember being involved in one workshop, which I think was about Mind Link. We had a moderate, factual discussion about involving service users. But at the end of it a social worker came up to me and said 'You're typically psychotic'. I mean, I was really shocked. It was like a head butt and meant that way.

We now have a kind of myth of partnership, 'oh yes we're all in partnership and we all should be in partnership and it is a good idea', but I think there's a myth to the extent that a lot of things that there is now a consensus about is not due to partnership, it's due to the fact that service users have been working in opposition, and service user involvement isn't just about working with people, it's sometimes about working against people. [In 2001 already, Peter had commented on the same theme: 'Whatever the slogans, real partnership is never easy. An important part of the survivor critique is about relationships with people in services and society. It is a mistake to accept the rhetoric of partnership at face value. This leaves us in a weak position to examine what is going on when we work with others. Instead, survivor organizations should be critical of the partnerships offered them, should decide for themselves what are the essential elements of partnership and be prepared to refuse to work with those who do not meet the criteria. The time to be afraid to turn down opportunities should be long past' ('Let's Be Real Partners!', *Community Care*, 15–21 November 2001)]

I think of 1985–1995 as a pioneering phase. One of the interesting issues is 'Did service user action really start in 1985?' The reason we've been celebrating this year, 21 years, is there is the perception that that's when things really started. I think in 1985–1986 significant things did happen. But it is also clear there were things going on before 1985, and some of those things fed into what happened after 1985. The Alleged Lunatics' Friend Society in 1845 was an advocacy organisation. It was service user controlled and it did have quite a lot of influence on the development of legislation in the mid-nineteenth century. The Mental Patients' Union (MPU), in the early 1970s, could probably be seen as the first service user involvement movement. Some people who were involved in the Mental Patients Union were also involved in the 1980s so there are direct links between the MPU and what happened in the early 1980s. Obviously there were also groups like Campaign Against Psychiatric Oppression and British Network of Alternatives to Psychiatry which were going in the early 1980s. They were quite small groups and there were not a large number of them. A lot of the ideas of these groups fed into Survivors Speak Out, which I helped to start, and Nottingham Advocacy Group (in 1986), and through them to the survivor movement as a whole.

It's worth knowing that there were things going on before 1985 and some of those things fed into what happened after 1985. On the other hand, I think in 1985–1986 significant things did happen. MIND has focused on the World Federation Conference held in Brighton in 1985, as a starting point. It's kind of ironic that they chose that, because the significant thing about that particular conference is there were hardly any service users from this country in it at all. In fact, I'm not sure that any service users from this country were officially invited. There were a number of service users from other countries invited and the real significance I think of that conference was that people suddenly asked 'Why aren't there any service users from the UK at this conference? We've got to do something about it because we know there are service users around who are taking action'. And that's what led to Survivors Speak Out being formed the following year. So I think the MIND conference in 1985 in Kensington was more significant, because it was the first national mental health conference where much of the programme was being run by service users, many of the workshops were being run by service users and service user organisations. Then in 1986 Survivors Speak Out was formed, the first national networking organisation. Nottingham Advocacy Group was also formed, which was extremely important because it promoted advocacy and patients' councils and shortly after that Mind Link, the service user network within national MIND and National Voices, a similar network within the National Schizophrenia Fellowship was formed. So I think it's true to say that in the mid 1980s service user action moved up a gear from what had happened before.

1985 to the early 1990s was about spreading the word. Going out to people and saying 'Look it is possible for service users to take action, this is why it's a good idea and this is how we can do it', and I think a lot of what was going on was people doing that, Survivors Speak Out, Nottingham Advocacy Group and other groups, going to local meetings around the country. One of the things that I remember that was exciting about this period, was that as Secretary of Survivors Speak Out I would get a letter from somebody, say in Wrexham, saying 'I'm a service user, I've heard about Survivors Speak Out, I want to set up a group', and then a couple of months later you'd be invited to go to a meeting in Wrexham to talk about developing service user action locally, and then maybe a few months later there would be a group in Wrexham. You could see little dots on the map and groups being set up where previously there had been nothing at all. So it was that kind of pioneering era.

What was going on was quite small scale compared to what happens nowadays. In 1990, there were about maybe 50 independent service user groups. Nowadays we're talking about more than 600 groups in England and Wales! We're also talking about quite a small degree of activity in 1990. Many of the groups were small, most of them were unfunded, many of them didn't have offices, the majority of them didn't have paid workers. This was the period before the user development worker. It was later in the 1990s that people were actually employed by various agencies to help set up user groups.

One of the striking things about the 1980s was that you knew people in a way you can't do now. It was quite possible if you were involved in a national organisation to feel that you knew a lot of the significant people who were involved in action around the country and nowadays things have got so enormous it isn't possible to know people in this way. Things have got so much more complicated, it's very difficult to know what to do to move things forward nationally. It's very difficult to know how to do things, because everything is so much more developed, more complex, whereas in those days it was much easier to say 'well this is what we need to do, and this is what we can do, and there are a lot of the things we can't do because we simply don't have the resources and won't be able to get them'. So I think in many ways things were a lot easier than they are nowadays. One of the things that has changed as well is expectations. In the early days we didn't have enormously high expectations of what could be done, we just thought, well we'll give it a go and see what happens, because it has never had been done before. Nowadays there are higher expectations of what you can achieve, what you should achieve. There are particularly high expectations from outside service user/survivor organisations and ideas about what service user/survivor organisations should be doing. So I think things have changed quite a lot since the pioneering phase.

If you look at the last ten years, what has happened is that service user involvement is now enshrined. It's not possible not to involve service users and those running the mental health system will not try to avoid involving service users.

Whether or not they actually listen to service users is another matter, but involving service users is an absolute necessity. I think you can see how in recent years voluntary mental health organisations like MIND or Together have pinned their flag to the flag pole of service user involvement. Service user involvement has become a big industry, many people are involved in it. We are involved in new areas of activity compared to the early 1990s. For example, research. Service user involvement in research is a huge area now. In the early 1990s it wasn't happening. So service users are involved across a huge area and people can now make a career in service user involvement. As a service user you can go out there and get paid work, sometimes quite well paid work. You can now pursue a career as a service user activist in a way that you couldn't ten years ago.

Another thing that has happened is specialisation. Because things have become so complex, there's a tendency for people to specialise in particular areas. In order to make any impact you have to spend all your time on self-harm, or on research, or on training and education. In some ways it fragments things and it's much more difficult to bring people together, because a lot of people are focused just on one particular area and may not be very aware of what's going on elsewhere. And I think that's one of the reasons there is a difficulty in getting a national voice for mental health service users, and difficulty in getting an overall sense of direction and cohesion. Because there is so much going on it is difficult to bring things together.

I think one of the things for me is that at least now there is an opportunity for people to take action in a way there wouldn't have been before. I think for somebody starting off their career as a mental health service user nowadays, they do have the opportunity to take action, to try to change things, to work with other service users, to speak out in public, to discuss their experiences with other people, to write, to teach, to do these things. Certainly, when I started off in the system in the 1960s, that was inconceivable. But I think it's very important that we do look at 'What are we trying to achieve? What are the things that we believe in, what are the principal things we believe in? What changes are we trying to achieve? How do we work together to achieve them better?' I think we do need to look not just at being here rather than nowhere but also at how we can make our presence more effective.

Thanks for listening.

3.12

'SECLUSION: THE BIGGER PICTURE' (2007)

Seclusion is a soft word for a harsh practice. For many people, talk of being in a secluded place will call up images of a quiet valley, a cottage in the shade of tall trees, sitting beside a stream. Somewhere that is peaceful and desirable. But seclusion in the context of mental health services is a quite different proposition. Here, seclusion is about bare rooms, closed doors, and abandonment. In mental health services seclusion means solitary confinement. If we used this latter term, it would help us better understand the real nature of what is going on.

A few years ago, I spoke at an international conference about my experiences in solitary confinement. An eminent mental health lawyer spoke immediately afterwards on the need to really define the costs and benefits of the practice. While accepting the importance of scientific evidence, I have always felt it might be more helpful to people confined in this way if it was assumed that the practice was likely to do some harm. This might make sensitive support for people emerging from solitary confinement more of a priority than it currently appears to be.

I believe the use of solitary confinement is sometimes justifiable. What angers me is the place it still holds in mental health services, and the way it is being regulated. In the early 1990s, there was talk of phasing out the practice in a few years. How far have we advanced towards that goal? The Mental Health Act Commission has been complaining regularly about hospitals' seclusion policies (inadequate, not updated, not following the Code of Practice etc.) ever since it came into existence. How much real difference has that made? There is certainly more talk about the issue in the mental health nursing profession than there used to be, but it is not clear that the recipients' experience of solitary confinement has improved very much. It is time the practice was covered by the Mental Health Act itself, and that the involvement of independent advocacy services in each episode became a legal necessity.

Of course, someone in great mental distress can also be put into solitary confinement in a police cell under section 136, and this has happened to me a number of times. I believe the practice should simply be outlawed. It is not necessary or desirable. It makes no therapeutic sense, is an abuse of human rights, and would hardly be tolerated in connection with any other group of disabled people in this country.

DOI: 10.4324/9781003636434-47

With all the money that has been injected into mental health services in recent years, why are we still using police cells as part of our crisis intervention response?

In 1992, the Reed Review of Health and Social Services for Disordered Offenders said: 'Police cells are not equipped for the detention of mentally disordered people whose presence there is likely to be deleterious to their mental health and may be degrading to their dignity'. Yet, fifteen years later, it is estimated that, on average, in each police force area, 328 people a year are being confined in police cells as 'a place of safety'. Home Office figures for 2004 showed that 20 out of 43 police forces in England and Wales were routinely using police cells in this way. If there is a problem here, and I don't believe the Reed Review's statement has ever been seriously challenged, we are certainly not moving very swiftly to solve it.

There are a number of reasons for this situation. Penny pinching is certainly important but underlying that is the low priority placed on the wants and needs of people in acute mental distress. Society does not know, and does not want to know, about the true nature of our crises, particularly if they involve 'psychotic' perceptions, thoughts and behaviour. Moreover, there is a basic lack of sympathy for our experiences in crisis that may not apply to other groups. Government and mental health workers' obsession with treatment compliance and the dogged and simplistic promotion of a 'they wouldn't have a crisis if they kept on taking their medication' line to the public is certainly not helping to give an accurate picture of what is going on, and why. Against this uninterested and uncomprehending background, it becomes easier for practices like solitary confinement to be seen as a tolerable, if not ideal, response to acute distress.

The solitary confinement of someone in great distress is a hazardous intervention – too hazardous to be undertaken by police officers. Such practice should cease. If I end up in solitary confinement in an acute ward again, I hope I will have a legal right to immediate advocacy and to proper support on returning to the day area. No mental health worker has ever spoken to me about what solitary confinement makes me feel about myself. Like many aspects of my crises over the last 40 years, it has simply been ignored. Changing the way we regulate solitary confinement is one thing. Salvaging the caring imagination is something else.

3.13

'PERSONAL ACCOUNT OF SECLUSION' (UNDATED)

I'm not able to forget the times I have been placed in solitary confinement. I almost began that statement with 'unfortunately', but I actually think it is not a good thing that people, either givers or receivers, should forget what goes on in the seclusion process. And forgiving is not forgetting – as all the good books say.

I've never asked to be locked up alone. Voluntary seclusion may be a good practice or a bad practice. It is certainly a quite different practice. If people in distress really want or need to be on their own, the psychiatric admission ward is probably the last place they should be seeking out.

Abandonment and punishment are the two main features of this sort of treatment in my estimation. There may be some symbolic meaning in the fact that my journeys into distress and confusion have occasionally climaxed with my lying alone on the floor of a small, bare room with very little clothing on. But there is not much comfort there. In my mind's eye, that isolation room always lies at the bottom of psychiatry's approach to asylum for me.

I remember standing many times squinting out of the window-slit in the door to see if anyone was there. I remember going on hunger strike during a prolonged spell of seclusion and having someone from the DHSS come in and interview me for benefit while I was just in underpants. What did all that add up to? I recall nurses blocking the doorway and saying calmly 'we're doing this to help you'. It sounds good but it never feels right.

How is it that people can be confined in police station cells for hours under section 136 before their distress is even attended to? Why is an independent advocate not called every time someone is placed into seclusion? Above all, why is there no clear right to counselling once we're let out? I have no easy answers to these questions and feelings. But somebody should be facing up to them.

DOI: 10.4324/9781003636434-48

3.14

'PEOPLE WITH MENTAL HEALTH PROBLEMS DON'T KNOW WHAT IS GOOD FOR THEM'

I am happy to oppose this proposition both as a mental health system survivor and as someone who has worked for many years as a nursery nurse. I would contend that the proposition is inimical both to people with a mental illness diagnosis and to good nursing practice.

It is good to have opportunity to debate the issue of differences. This is particularly important at a time when we are moving towards community care. How are people with mental health problems different from others? How are they different from other disabled people?

As it stands, the proposition is obviously too sweeping. People with mental health problems are a huge group and includes people with both 'neurotic' and 'psychotic' problems. Clearly, many of them will have every ability to know what is good for them. I would happily argue against any suggestion that people with 'psychotic problems' do not know what is good for them, but this proposition is much broader even than that.

I am not denying that people with mental health problems will sometimes not know what is good for them but contend that this is true of all human beings. The proposition is not a useful distinction between this group and other groups.

The proposition implies that there is a permanent condition of not knowing here. This overlooks the episodic nature of madness and the fact that insight, even in the psychiatric version, can and should be seen as a dynamic possibility. In psychiatric care, insight and disagreements over treatment are often confused together. They should be distinguished.

I contend that most people with mental health problems know what is good for them and are trying to achieve those goals. We should not confuse a failure to achieve those goods with an inability to know what they are.

Unpublished notes for a presentation opposing this proposition.

                                    DOI: 10.4324/9781003636434-49

Drug treatment is often used as an example of where people with mental health problems do not know what is good for them. In fact, it is often very difficult to make clear and rational decisions around drug taking. It is difficult to balance positive and negative effects. Not taking a psychiatric drug may be a most rational choice. Moreover, we should not forget the high numbers of people without a mental illness diagnosis who do not continue with the medications prescribed for them.

If we support the proposition, we must confront the reasons why we seek to involve this group in discussions about mental health services, even as consumers. If we really feel they do not know what is good for them, what sort of hypocrisy inspires efforts at user involvement?

We would also have to account for the uncomfortable reality that many people value self-help approaches and seem convinced that people with similar experiences do have particular contributions to make, whether or not the outcomes are significantly different as a result. Is this just communal self-delusion?

I would contend that people with mental health problems not only know what is good for them but know what good itself is. This awareness of where the good is, and where they stand in relation to it, following a mental illness diagnosis, lies behind much of the long-term psychological distress this group experiences.

In conclusion, I would like to cite two quotations from Michael Ignatieff:

> 'There are few presumptions in human relations more dangerous than the idea that one knows what another human being needs better than they do themselves'
>
> (*The Needs of Strangers*, p.11)

and:

> 'The arrogation of the right by doctors to define the needs of their patients, of social workers to administer the needs of their clients … is in all cases a warrant for abuse.'
>
> (*The Needs of Strangers*, p.11)

I believe that the proposition is neither accurate nor useful. It makes quite the wrong kind of presumptions about people with mental health problems. Even if there were more truth in it, it would be a bad basis on which to proceed into a future of better care. I ask you to oppose this proposition.

Reference

Ignatieff, Michael (1984) *The Needs of Strangers*. London: Chatto & Windus, The Hogarth Press.

3.15

'SPEAKING FOR OURSELVES'

'I first became involved in action by mental health system users/survivors in the UK in the mid-1980s. At that time the range of activity was extending considerably and I would be actively involved until at least the end of the century. The three groups I was most involved in were Survivors Speak Out, founded in 1986; Survivors' Poetry, founded in 1991, and Survivors' History Group, founded in 2005.

Survivors Speak Out was my prime focus from 1986 to 1996, so much so that I limited my activity in Survivors Poetry within 18 months of being a founder member. There was not enough time for me to devote to the two groups and I felt Survivors Speak Out had my first loyalty. After 1996, I was not involved in a group but spent my energies as a freelance trainer of mental health workers. Then, in 2005, I became a founder member of Survivors History Group, a gathering of mental health system survivors interested in ensuring they should write and research their own histories. This is the only group I am still involved in.

Any discussion of what we call ourselves must start and end in the principle of self-definition. People must always be able to choose how they describe themselves and have that respected. This is important whether they want to call themselves consumers, service users, survivors, schizophrenics, anorexics or the mentally ill. We have been burdened for too long with alien names. We must not alienate others by calling them names they do not own. Having said that, I do have a clear preference of term – mental health system survivor. First of all, I feel that survivor (I am surviving, not I have survived) is a positive term and points rightly to the obstacle course of the mental health system that I am endeavouring to survive. But, equally important, it is not a question of mental health services or psychiatry alone. These are important, and can be oppressive, but they are part of a wider system, a socio-political system that is founded on prejudices and misunderstandings of people diagnosed with so-called mental disorders. I feel most comfortable thinking of my life in relation to a mental health system. It points to the true nature of my dilemma in a way "psychiatric" survivor or mental health service survivor does not.

The text of an email interview that Peter contributed in 2022 to The Routledge International Handbook of Mad Studies, Edited by Peter Beresford and Jasna Russo © 2022 by Routledge. Reproduced by permission of Taylor & Francis Group.

DOI: 10.4324/9781003636434-50

The main nature of my action has been in three areas. These have been, first, the organisation and activities of the UK networking group Survivors Speak Out (1986 to 1996). Second, freelance training with mental health workers – especially clinical psychologists, social workers and mental health nurses, with a particular focus on the lived experience of mental health system survivors; the reform of the 1983 Mental Health Act; and work on the role and function of mental health nurses. Third, and finally, the writing of numerous chapters, usually on the "service user/survivor movement" and allied topics, in various mental health textbooks and including regular articles and book reviews in *OpenMind*, the bi-monthly and now much-missed magazine of MIND (formerly the National Association of Mental Health) which gave mental health system survivor activists an unparalleled voice for many years.

Much of this work was time-consuming. Most of it was poorly paid if paid at all. I believe my last three years' work at Survivors Speak Out led me to "burn out". Instead of planning new campaigns or publications like the very successful "Self Harm – From Personal Perspectives", I was addressing envelopes, dealing with membership fees, answering personal correspondence and other administrative tasks. The eventual arrival of paid workers brought many managerial challenges. Maintaining the infrastructure of action groups was often less enjoyable than action itself. A fact which may help explain why some groups found it hard to continue long term.

My areas of action included working with mental health system survivors and working with mental health workers. With both groups, I emphasized the importance of self-advocacy – individuals and groups speaking and acting for change on their own terms. This made clear, at the outset, the possibilities of action, of people being the masters of their own destiny. It also encouraged diversity rather than agreed agendas and platforms. The aim was not to replace one dominant force (psychiatry) with another – a monocultural survivor movement.

Alongside self-advocacy, speaking and acting for yourself, with particular relevance to services, was advocacy – an innovation of the 1980s. The survivor movement championed the right of service users to have another person support them in voicing their wants and needs or to speak up on their behalf completely. As a freelance trainer, I promoted the understanding and practical application of both these concepts. Unfortunately, the very real gain in life choices that resulted was mystified by the false rhetoric of "user empowerment" which suggested much more was going on than was actually the case. It is true that service users had more control over their lives, within and outside the system, but they certainly were not equal. People with a diagnosis of a so-called "mental disorder" remain, as ever, a disempowered rather than an empowered group.

The United Nations Convention for the Rights of People with Disabilities (UN CRPD) has not really played a part, or been relevant, to me and my work. I will be very surprised if the compulsion-free care and treatment the UN CRPD appears to envisage will be introduced in the UK in the foreseeable future. Developments seem to be going in the opposite direction with more, not less, compulsory detention and treatment. It has taken 37 years to outlaw the use of police station cells as places of safety under Section 136 of the 1983 Mental Health Act. If a minor but vital change of this kind is so long in coming, the sweeping changes the UN CPRD encourages seem unlikely to arrive any time soon.

In my view, there are three main aspects of our first-hand knowledge. First, knowledge of living in, and receiving, mental health services. Secondly, living with mental distress in society. Finally, first-hand knowledge of the interior experience of distress (the "madness experience"). These are of varying interest to service providers. They are enthusiastic about service users as consumers, not particularly interested in the experience of living in society with mental distress, and often uninterested or hostile to first-hand and alternative accounts of distress.

The 1990s were the era of "user involvement" when activists were first invited to contribute their knowledge to community care plans. At the same time, they told their life stories in training mental health workers.

By the end of the decade, the service user as conveyor of "consumer expertise" was widely accepted. At the same time, another rather different development had been taking place. A number of groups emerged using their first-hand understandings of mental distress to put forward alternatives. The Hearing Voices Network (HVN) and the National Self Harm Network (NSHN) are good example of these. These groups were radical and their challenge to psychiatric orthodoxy was rooted in first-hand knowledge. Their work helped first-hand understanding to gain a new value.

First-hand knowledge does now have a new respectability. But it is not entirely a rosy picture. Professionally derived knowledge is still regularly given a higher value than our first-hand knowledge. Survivor-led research is not respected in the way other research is. It would be good to see our knowledge existing on a level playing field with professional knowledge. It would also be good to see more emphasis on our first-hand knowledge of living with distress in society, and to see our experience being considered alongside that of other disabled people. Above all else, our first-hand knowledge of the interior experience of mental distress/madness deserves to hold a central place whenever psychiatry is taught.

I see psychiatry in the United Kingdom as a mechanism of social control. Individuals are controlled by being compulsorily detained and "treated" often for considerable periods. Psychiatry is at the heart of a system that creates a second class of citizens; people who can be treated differently, even if they have retained the capacity to make decisions. It concentrates on the individual pathology of these people, suggesting that they are incompetent and "do not know what is in their best interests". Psychiatry acts conservatively, reinforcing social prejudice and fitting its recipients into the status quo, rather than trying to change their social environment. While ostensibly looking only to help the distressed, psychiatry is in fact moulding them for roles as the disempowered.

The big question for the survivor movement is whether to try to improve psychiatry or to build alternatives to it. In the UK, the movement has by and large sought to improve psychiatry, while leaving the deeper problem virtually untouched.

In this way they have achieved some important positive change without fundamentally challenging psychiatry as a potentially oppressive practice. In the 1980s there was a constant challenge to psychiatry as a form of social control, but that seems to have receded now. It could be claimed that the survivor movement has been co-opted into the mental health system and its challenge fundamentally blunted. The more radical demands of activists have been almost completely resisted. Whatever its history, by and large the survivor movement has become a reformist enterprise.

Unfortunately, the emergence of Mad Studies coincided with my stepping back from involvement in the survivor movement. In short, I know too little of Mad Studies to make meaningful comments. Having said that, any survivor-controlled initiative that provides a radical critique of psychiatry, and seeks to build alternatives to it, would have my support. Whether Mad Studies does those things, will have to be for others to judge.'

Part 4

Big Red and Afterwords

4.00

BIG RED

As mentioned earlier, in the 1980s Peter was also experimenting with writing for young children. To provide a taste of his creations from this period, we reproduce here his vivid and wittily-observed story Big Red.

Angus and Colin went down to the chip shop for their supper. On the way home they took a shortcut through the park along the street with the big red wall.

As they walked past, they thought they could hear a huffling* sound.
"I think we are being followed," said Angus.
They looked behind them.
A big red monster had come out of the wall and was walking after them.

They walked a little faster.
The huffling noise came after them just as fast.
Angus stopped and looked at the monster. The monster was looking at the bag in Colin's hand.
"I think it wants one of your chips," said Angus.

The red monster stretched his long neck over Colin's shoulder and took the bag of chips.
After huffling once or twice it spat the bag out onto the pavement.
"Perhaps it doesn't like vinegar," said Angus.
"I don't care," said Colin. "I'm going to take him home."

"What do you mean take him home? What will your mother say?"
"He seems to be friendly," Colin replied. "Besides, my mother likes animals she said to herself."
Angus was too surprised to speak, but he was very glad he didn't live in the same block of flats as Colin.

---

*huffle, a sudden gust of wind, or the sound made by this, [OED 1889]

DOI: 10.4324/9781003636434-52

By the time they had reached the entrance to the flats, Colin had decided to call the monster Big Red. Emily Biscuit, who knew everything, was standing waiting for the lift. Colin went up behind her and said, "This is my new pet, Big Red. Would you like to meet him?" Emily turned round. She was so surprised that she fell over. Big Red picked her up and put her back down on her feet.

"I'll have to go now," said Angus. "How are you going to get Big Red upstairs? He's too big to fit inside the lift."
"We'll walk upstairs. I'm sure he can squeeze up that way."
"OK then." Angus began to run off home. Halfway across the yard he turned round and shouted, "See you tomorrow, Colin. And be careful."

Big Red stuck his head and neck out low and walked very slowly and carefully. With Colin leading him he was just able to climb upstairs.
Emily Biscuit watched from the ground floor.
"I really have seen everything now," she muttered.

Colin and Big Red passed Mrs McPherson coming down.
"Good evening, Colin and good evening to your friend," she said and walked down without stopping.
Everything was going well.

When they reached the flat, Colin's Mum came to the door.
"This is my new pet, Mum. Can I keep him?"
Mum looked at Big Red.
"You had better bring him in. But he'll have to eat fish, same as the cat."

Colin went into the sitting room and introduced Big Red to everyone. There was Maureen, the twins, Uncle Alec and Granny O'Grady. "We're watching the telly, so keep your mouth shut," said Uncle Alec. When Big Red lay down, Colin and the twins climbed up and sat on him. So mum was able to sit on the sofa for the first time for years.

That night Colin was woken up by the moonshine. He went to see how Big Red was. He was asleep on the carpet with his head resting on the television set and his tail hanging out of the window. They would have great times tomorrow!

* *

Next morning, they went down to the adventure playground. The children put ladders up against Big Red, measured how long and how tall he was, investigated the gaps in his feet and the space inside his ears. They slid down Big Red's back into the paddling pool and made him lie down in the water to form a desert island. It was a highly successful day.

Big Red became well known in the housing estate. Colin and Angus would take him out for long walks around the park when Murphy the park keeper was away

home for his tea. They didn't go out on the main streets just in case. But nobody really seemed to notice. "I think you've cracked it, Colin," Angus said.
"Cracked what?"
"Keeping a monster in a block of flats."

Everyone liked Big Red.
Emily Biscuit came up to the flat one morning with a big book.
"I think he's a gigantocus, Colin."
They looked at the picture in the book. It certainly seemed like Big Red. They showed the picture to Big Red, but he picked the book up and swallowed it whole.
"Does that mean Yes or No?" asked Colin.

Mrs MacPherson kept coming down with sponge cakes for Big Red. "It's no bother," she told Colin's mum, "It's nice to have someone who appreciates my cooking."
Colin's mum was happy she could hang the twin's nappies out to dry on Big Red and not have to climb all the way down to the drying green.

One evening, Colin and Angus took Big Red to the chip shop. They went past the red wall, but the monster didn't seem to notice. Mrs MacPhail who owned the chip shop was delighted to meet Big Red. "If you get him to stand just outside the door, he'll bring in more customers and you can have as many chips as you want for nothing."
So they went down every night for half an hour. Mrs MacPhail sold so much that she ran out of potatoes.

Only Uncle Alec was unhappy. He sat in front of the television and told Colin what the facts were. "The thing is son, everything has its proper place in this world. You'll have to learn that. I'm not saying you're doing wrong. But I'm not sure that a flat on the 13th floor is the proper place for a monster." "Why not Uncle Alec?" Colin asked. "Because. Because it's never been done before, son."

That night Colin couldn't sleep. He went to the window and looked out over the housing estate. There were four towers of flats and the lights of the city behind them. He wondered how many Uncle Alecs there were out there. He began to count all the lights he could see. Suddenly he had a terrible sinking feeling in his stomach.

****

Next morning there was a loud knocking on the door. Colin went out and opened it. There was a man standing there, dressed all in gray with a small black hat on his head. "Who are you?" Colin asked. "I am an official," the man said, and he handed Colin a little card. On it was written in big letters THIS MAN IS AN OFFICIAL and besides the words a picture of a man all in gray with a small black hat on his head. "What is an official?", Colin asked. "That's none of your business, son. I want to speak to your mother."

They went into the kitchen. Colin's mom was there. So was Big Red. The man took his hat off and hung it on Big Red's head. "I want to talk to you about this animal, there's been complaints." Colin's mum sat down and blew her nose. "Go on then. I'm listening." "Not in front of these two," the man said without looking at Colin and Big Red. "This is official business."

And so Colin sat in the room outside with Big Red and the twins. He could hear the man talking in the kitchen. It went on and on. Colin realized that the game was up. After a while Big Red began to eat the official's small black hat. Very slowly and carefully. By the time the man came out, the hat was all gone. "Good day to you," said the official. "And to you mister," Colin replied. "I'm afraid this animal has eaten your hat." The official began to speak, then looked at Big Red and changed his mind. He went out and closed the front door very hard.

Colin's mum made a cup of tea and sat down to tell him the bad news. There had been complaints. Mrs MacPhail had sold so many chips that all the other chip shops were jealous. People from across the other side of the city were coming over to Mrs MacPhail's just because it was where the monster was.

Granny O'Grady had been using Big Red's neck as a quick way of getting down from the 2nd floor and Mr. O'Grady didn't like it. Murphy the park keeper was upset that people kept telling him that there was a monster in his park, and he had never seen it.

"But that's not much bad," Colin complained. "I know you're right," his mum said. "But that's not the real reason. It's his colour that's the trouble. It's not usual for an animal you see. The man says he might be confused with a post box or a fire engine. It could have unfortunate consequences."

Colin thought of the gray concrete flats with their dark damp patches where the rain ran down. He thought of Big Red standing in the middle with children climbing all over him. He remembered what Uncle Alec said. Officials and monsters just don't mix.

As a last chance he said, "What about goldfish mum, they're red?" "I know son. The man said if we wanted to claim Big Red was a goldfish he'd have to live in a bowl. He'd not take to that. I'm afraid we're beaten this time. That's life."

Colin went into the bedroom. He couldn't think of anything that was less than life. Particularly for Big Red.
What would happen to him? Colin remembered the skeletons in the animal museum, surrounded by notice boards and fire buckets. Big Red certainly wasn't going to end up there. He would not let the officials get him.

Next morning at half-past nine Colin donated Big Red to the adventure playground. MacSweeney the playworker was delighted.
"But is he properly trained?"
"Yes, he is," Colin replied, "And he likes his chips with vinegar."
"Excellent," said MacSweeney. "We have important visitors tomorrow. This should impress them."

All day, Colin and Angus taught Big Red to stand very still and not huffle too much. Emily Biscuit came to help them.
"This is going to be the greatest escape story ever," she said.

The following morning, the sun was shining in a blue sky. Big Red looked bigger and redder than ever. The mayor arrived at the playground gate. He had a golden chain around his neck and a little man in a white jacket following beside him writing things in a book.
"Watch out for the wee man with the book," Colin told Angus, "He looks like an official."

Big Red stood as still as a dinosaur in the Museum. The mayor leant against his front leg and said, "Magnificent, so lifelike!"
MacSweeney said, "Yes and it's all made out of wire and papier mache, your honour!" "Really?" replied the mayor and went off to the playhut for something to drink.

Then the man with the notebook took a large rubber stamp out of his back pocket and pressed it against Big Red's leg. Big Red didn't move a muscle. When the man had gone, they all crept back to look. There was a black mark on Big Red saying OFFICIAL SEAL OF APPROVAL.
"What does that mean?" Colin asked.
"It means they can never get rid of Big Red now," said Emily Biscuit.
"It means you've done it Colin. You've won!"

And that was the truth of it. When the first official went back to Colin's flat, there was no monster. Uncle Alec saw him off. Colin's mum knew something funny had been going on, but she knew better than to ask what had happened to Big Red.

And as for Big Red, he was big enough to look over the edge of the playground wall and tease people in the street, and clever enough to stand completely still whenever anyone who looked like an official was near.

Word spread. So, the adventure playground was always busy, and whenever it was cold and gray, Colin and Angus and the other children would buy chips and sit out with Big Red. And sometimes they would check the black mark on his leg and polish it up so that it did not fade away. And then they would sit in the mud, surrounded by chip packets, and laugh until their buttons started to pop.

The End.

4.01

Reflecting on Peter:
The Editors

In conclusion, it may be helpful to locate Peter's work and achievements in the current mental health landscape. How do they appear today and what value may they have looking forward? In the first of three afterwords, we contribute a brief assessment ourselves. This is followed by invited commentaries from two current mental health system survivors, both of them vocal and active in distinctive ways, Sarah Carr and Colin King.

Afterword 1 by the editors

The time when Peter was in his prime, and the mental health survivor movement was at its apogee, is significantly different from the current moment. This is not to glamourise the past and dismiss valuable developments that may be happening today. In the current cultural climate, for example, there is unquestionably increased openness about struggles, a re-kindling of Mad Pride activities post-pandemic, an increased appreciation and understanding of intersectionality and of the value of diverse voices and approaches.

All the same, this is now a time shaped by the violence of austerity[1] under the guise of welfare reform where claimants live under the threat of constant benefits reassessments, mental health survivors and others are frequently targeted as parasites and a drain on the taxpayer and dwell in palpable fear of a 'hostile environment' consuming minds and lives (Cooper and Whyte, 2017). Among others, China Mills has documented welfare state violence by centring the resistance of people with lived experience of the welfare system (Mills, 2018; see also Pring, 2024). Peter Campbell was acutely aware of these developments and lent his support to resistance that was taking place (2020, 2022).

The kinds of people who once may have fought for radical changes in the mental health system are now having to put their energy into fighting for any treatment at all. Many people are fearful of questioning treatment due to the risk of being discharged for non-compliance and left with nothing (and with no supporting evidence

DOI: 10.4324/9781003636434-53

for benefits). Some people may also be taking medications that don't help, or make their conditions worse, due to the risk of a benefit assessor saying that they can't be that bad if they aren't on many medications. The changes and scarcity in mental health treatment and charity provision (day wards and centres or drop in services exist no more) reduce the opportunities for people to meet and organise or question the legitimacy or use of the labels and treatments on offer. The result is that issues and lives are inordinately at risk of remaining individualised.

Under these conditions, it is hard to imagine how broad collective action like *Survivors Speak Out* could be possible today. If you are seen to be able to organise and work in this way, how can you also be seen to be eligible for state support in a culture where the assumption is you are a fraud? This inevitably limits the possibilities, and range, of service users able to write, campaign or add their voice to debates in the way that Peter Campbell so compellingly did over his life. The scope and ambition of his work – and of the survivor movement in general – is thus ever more vital to preserve and pay attention to. The hope and imagination to envision and work towards another way of doing things, the possibility of solidarity and community, the creativity and humour, as well as the clear-sighted critique and advocacy, are all vital to draw on in ongoing and future struggles.

Note

1 This term is borrowed from *The Violence of Austerity,* Cooper, Vickie and Whyte, David (eds), Pluto Press, 2017.

References

Campbell, Peter (2020) 'Preface by Peter Campbell' In Peter Barham, *Closing the Asylum: The Mental Patient in Modern Society*, third edition, with a preface by Peter Campbell. London: Process Press Ltd.
Campbell, Peter [3.15 (2022)] 'Speaking for Ourselves'.
Cooper, Vickie and Whyte, David eds. (2017) *The Violence of Austerity.* London: Pluto Press.
Mills, China (2018) 'Dead people don't claim': a psychopolitical autopsy of UK austerity suicides', *Critical Social Policy*, Vol. 38, pp. 302–322.
Pring, John (2024) *The Department: How a Violent Government Bureaucracy Killed Hundreds and Hid the Evidence*. London: Pluto Press.

4.02

AFTERWORD 2 BY DR. SARAH CARR FRSA, SURVIVOR RESEARCHER AND SERVICE USER INVOLVEMENT CHAMPION

As a founder and leader of the survivor movement, Peter's activism was undoubtedly political, but he was also a philosophical activist. Through his writings he has bequeathed us deeper philosophical insight into our personal and communal experiences.

In 'Therapeutica – Chinks in the Armour' [1.05], Peter describes the healing challenge of human encounters in a therapeutic community and the importance of listening to both fellow survivors and staff. We can learn a great deal from his ability to listen, particularly his capacity to hear and interpret silence. In his calm critique of psychiatry, Peter highlights its silencing effect. He argues that it imposes the view that mental distress is a 'meaningless disease' – there is no interest or discussion, no value placed on the 'patient' perspective. Psychiatry's lack of curiosity results in the silencing of those who, in Peter's case, experience what is called psychosis. But, as his body of work shows, he did not remain silent. In 'Valuing Psychosis' [2.14] he says, 'let's start working to cut out the silence'. He shares with us his journey to finding his own voice and then to empowering others to have a voice, but also to listen.

In 'Valuing Psychosis' [2.14], Peter also emphasises the point that 'the major obstacle to individuals finding their own value for psychosis is psychiatry itself'. For him, survivors are not 'victims of chronic illness', but those of philosophies that cannot encompass the complexities of madness, distress and altered states. He reminds us that psychiatry cannot necessarily help us find meaning in 'interior experiences' or explore the external factors that influence mental distress. I and countless others have struggled with psychiatric opinions about personal distress. When I heard voices, the psychiatrist was not equipped to help me work out what I was experiencing. According to her, my voices were 'pseudo hallucinations', and while I did not believe the voices came from external sources, they were still real to me. My so-called 'insight' resulted in the invalidation of my interior experiences,

    DOI: 10.4324/9781003636434-54

and I was left to make sense of them myself. I owe a great deal to Peter because I wasn't alone in my endeavour and was able to draw on the wisdom of survivor elders who had been there before me.

As his writings attest, Peter developed a strong belief in his own understanding and gave other survivors the means to believe in theirs. By encountering his work, we come to understand the injurious limitations of psychiatric concepts and treatment, and what these do to us as human beings, individually and collectively. We also come to understand the power of our knowledge.

4.03

AFTERWORD 3 BY COLIN KING, BLACK SURVIVOR RESEARCH ACTIVIST AND FOUNDER OF THE *WHITENESS AND RACE EQUALITY NETWORK*

Speaking for myself as a black racialized misdiagnosed male, Peter's case reso-nates. I empathise and celebrate his bravery, his resilience and embrace his position as an activist for change in relation to the historical dehumanization he endured. He captures vividly the legacy of slavery, a modern Drapetomania, across lines of race and class as a poet and a writer from a similar period in which I was savagely brutalized and medicalized in the journey from a mental health enslaved prisoner to become an agent of the state as a mental health practitioner. Consequently, the essential quality and uniqueness of this book is that it legitimizes the experiences, words and creativity of Peter as a lived experience that is authentically epistemo-logical centred. It challenges the mistruth of current diagnostic frameworks that represent the illusions and forms of cultural entrapment. Peter's story, his work and his life are groundbreaking and a liberation of the black voice during a similar period in which schizophrenia has become a black disease and has been trans-formed into a formula for castration, murder and restraint. A mental health legisla-tion is based on criminalization, cost-effectiveness and the politics of the black body as a medical commodity of control.

Peter gives permission to declare your passion as a mental health warrior, as a combat for a new morality and a new model of humanity, in my journey from being labelled educationally subnormal, schizophrenic, to suffer prison and hos-pital admissions within a historical dominance of whiteness. A whiteness that is both medically intrusive and personally a psychosis of destruction. Whilst suicide is often considered a form of total escapism, Peter motivates a new approach to systems of whiteness as the need to consider institutional suicide inside white-ness. The whiteness in which research of race is a deception of a reality main-tained through legal and social policies: mental health reform bill, advance choice to death, a culture of neglect and deception. Peter not only in his academic bravery,

 DOI: 10.4324/9781003636434-55

but his sense of seeing and challenging injustice represents marginalized prisoners within the illegitimacy of mental health as a biologically misinformed science of mass destruction. He has become a saviour in challenging the politics of mental health policy, the wards of death, and the neo-liberal devastation of health inequalities in modern Britain. Peter's oratory, his declaration of his first-person despair represents a passage and a revelation of mental health as ideological and repressive framework. He articulates the potential for whiteness to use its privilege, its entitlement to challenge and change a system that permits the collusive racialized relationship between mental health as political structure of a global racism.

I feel Peter's energy through his biography and life, his personal commitment towards radical ethical dismantling of a mental health system that contributed towards my cultural death, entrapment and worthlessness. He has resurrected my mission and my vision through my chapter 'They diagnosed me a schizophrenic when I was just a Gemini' (2006) to ensure the legacy of Peter is enshrined and celebrated.

Reference

King, Colin (2006) 'They diagnosed me a schizophrenic when I was just a Gemini. "The other side of madness"'. In Man Cheung Chung, Bill Fulford and George Graham (Eds.) *Reconceiving Schizophrenia*, International Perspectives in Philosophy & Psychiatry, Oxford: Oxford University Press, online edition Oxford Academic.

4.04

ACKNOWLEDGEMENTS

We are hugely grateful to Peter's surviving brother Lennox Campbell and other members of the Campbell family for their unflagging support of this project and for granting us permission to reproduce all of Peter's unpublished writings.

We are honoured to be able to publish this book under the acclaimed book series of the International Society for Psychological and Social Approaches to Psychosis [ISPS] and we are very grateful to the ISPS series editor, Dr Anna Lavis, for her guidance and support in the completion of this work.

We would like to thank Louise R. Pembroke and Professor Barbara Taylor for their stimulating forewords and for responding readily to us when we have reached out to them over the past two years.

Though, sadly, owing to his declining health Andrew Roberts was unable to involve himself directly in bringing this collection to fruition, his presence hovers over everything that we have done and we wish to thank him for his friendship, and to acknowledge the huge debt that we owe him, over many years in assembling an incomparable resource of mental health survivor-related material that will, we anticipate, continue to inspire and support generations to come.

Many of Peter Campbell's friends have been supportive over the three years since Peter died but we want to single out particularly Thurstine Basset and Hel Spandler for their thoughtful comments and reflections and for making themselves available to us when we needed them, together with James Campbell, Alison Faulkner, Jim Reed, Diana Rose and Nikolas Rose.

Our thanks to Anne E. Plumb in Manchester for her friendly help with our inquiries and for facilitating access to the 'Ear to the Ground' archive, her unparalleled personal archive collection in mental health, in conjunction with Manchester Libraries, Information and Archives, Manchester City Council.

Our warm thanks to Nat Fonnesu for supplying, and permitting us to use, her photograph of Peter performing 'The Mental Marching Band'.

Our thanks to everyone at Bishopsgate Institute Archives and Collection Centre where Peter Campbell's archives are held, notably Stefan Dickers, Special Collections & Archives Manager, and Robyn Nightingale, who also archived Andrew

DOI: 10.4324/9781003636434-56

Roberts's materials, also Ceri, Niamh, Rachel and Colleen, archive staff who helped facilitate access for Ker to the stores etc.

Our gratitude to all those individuals and bodies who have given us permission to reproduce interviews or articles by Peter that fell within their domains, notably the National Sound Archive at the British Library for the 'Testimony 2000' interview and Johnny Bird at MIND publications for the right to reproduce Peter's articles from *OpenMind* magazine: copyright MIND, www.mind.org.uk.

Our warm thanks to Emily Johns and Susan Johns from Hearing Eye Press for their interest and support for our project and for the inclusion of two of Peter's poems, 'The Mental Marching Band' and 'Crisis Advocate', and a verse from 'Drugtime Cowboy Joe' from the Hearing Eye collection '*Brown Linoleum Green Lawns*' (2006).

Our very warm thanks, lastly, to Dr Sarah Carr and to Colin King for their thoughtful contributions, produced at very short notice, for the Afterwords.

4.05

RESOURCES

Mental Health Testimony Archive, which includes Peter Campbell's 2000 Testimony interview, accessible to view at the British Library, www.bl.uk., ref: C905/50.

Peter Campbell Legacy Project [PCLP] Archive, accessible at the Bishopsgate Institute.

Also at the Bishopsgate Institute, Survivors' Network Archives, collections donated by Andrew Roberts,

Andrew Roberts's website and archive: http://studymore.org.uk/

Asylum, the radical mental health magazine, www.asylummagazine.org

Disability News Service, run by John Pring, a disabled journalist who has been reporting on disability issues for nearly 25 years, www.disabilitynewsservice.com

International Society for Psychological and Social Approaches to Psychosis [ISPS], www.isps.org, https://isps.org/isps-book-series/

Concord Media, a major educational distributor of audio-visual material on mental health issues, notably the film of '*We're Not Mad, We're Angry' (1986)* [2.02], https://www.concordmedia.org.uk/products/were-not-mad-were-angry-483/

Ear to the Ground, Survivor, service user, mad identified (SSUMI+) and ally voices, organisations and action in the UK 1971–2010, catalogue of a personal archive collection in mental health by Anne E. Plumb, TBR Imprint, Manchester 2022.

Hearing Eye, the publisher of Peter Campbell's poetry collection *Brown Linoleum Green Lawns* (2006), a small independent press with a rich history and a vibrant website at: www.hearingeye.org

DOI: 10.4324/9781003636434-57

INDEX

Note: Page numbers in *italics* refer to illustrations.

workers are invested in keeping users inferior and passive 127; *Big Red.* (story) 213–217; Cambridge Simon Community 21; *Camden Mental Health Consortium* xxxvi; can never escape the memory of severe breakdown, 26; CAPO *(Campaign Against Psychiatric Oppression)* xxxvi; as a 'career psychotic', a veteran of the mental health system xxiv; central element in PC's life, loss of, and attempts to re-establish, self-control xxvii, 92–98; creative writing xxix–xxxi; early education 11, 19–21; developing sense (1971) that something was permanently amiss 23; early life xxxvi, 10–11; ECT as a radicalising experience 182; emphatic about owning and integrating his own madness and distress xxvi; experience of being detained on a Section of the Mental Health Act 141; family 10–11; feels he is a failure but at deep level enjoys task of return 164; first crisis xxv; first decades of his mental health career xxv; First in History 22; Freudian interpretation of life 17; at Fulbourn Hospital, Cambridge 24; having a career in the mental health system 117,120; how has he been affected by psychiatrists' assertions that the contents of psychosis are meaningless? 119; intellectual ability 17–18; at Jesus College, Cambridge xxv, 10–11; locating PC's work and achievements in the current mental health landscape 218–222; in Richmond Fellowship therapeutic community 47–53; at Royal Dundee Liff Hospital & discharge 13–16, 17–18; in West Park hospital Epsom 44–45; memory of a padded cell on a locked ward 44; memory of two asylum admissions as gross insult to his human rights 32; *Mental Health Testimony Archive*, with interview by PC, 61; in the 1970s often felt that his crises would destroy him 128; in North Kensington house 48; objects to way in which power is stripped from him 94; PC's key insights xxviii–xxix; psychiatric orthodoxy, a stern critic of xxvi; psychiatric system survivor movement xxii, 21; questions the psychiatric belief that he has a psychotic element in his make-up and needs an anti-psychotic drug for life 191; self-advocacy xxvii–xxix; survivor movement xxix–xxxi; Survivors History Group, founder member 206

CAPO *see* Campaign Against Psychiatric Oppression

care and control 155

career 89

Care Management 124

Care Programme Approach (CPA) 123–124; service user's perspective 122–127

Carr, Sarah 218, 220–221

cartoons by Niall, 'Melvin Menz' *81–83*

casual observation 34

casualty staff 28

chemotherapy 17; controlling power of 53–55; thanks to, 'the so-called mentally ill will win in the end' 55, 187–192

chloral hydrate 53

chlorpromazine 31–32, 188

civil rights legislation 160

Clunis, Christopher 124

Cohen, Bruce M.Z. xxiii

coma 155

Coming Out of the Closet' (*Testimony* 2000) 153–154

Common Concerns Conference 197

Community Care Act, 1990 158

confusion 35

Conolly, John 61

constitutional inadequacy xxiii

consultant interview 71–73

containment 163–164

'Control in the Community' (Campbell) 155–156

Cooper, David xxxvi

counsellors 47

criminalization 222

crisis care, failings of xxvi, 104–106, 162–164; 'finding myself alone at 1.30 a.m., contemplating my own disintegration' 28

crisis prevention 109

Crossley, Nick xxiii

Cyrene Community 22

degrees of self-advocacy 100–103

degrees of unreality 19

de Nerval, Gerard 19

of illness in its psychiatric context 52;
those excluded from 40; power fields
of history, precarious lives that are
immersed in xxiii
powerlessness 32; the dominant condition
of the admission ward dweller 39; of the
patient within a bureaucratic system 95;
sustained by attitudes maintaining that
the 'mentally ill' are negatively different
from their fellow human beings 103;
system demands that patients admit to
and hand themselves over to experts 93
priadel 63
professional workers, power of 39, 46–47
psyche, vicissitudes of xxiii
psychiatric admission ward 94
psychiatric asylums xvii–xviii, xxvi, 13, 61,
103, 146, 155–157, 160, 169, 172–174
psychiatric care 14, 35
psychiatric drugs 53–56, 187–192, 205
psychiatric imagination 105
psychiatric system survivor movement
xxii
psychiatric wards 36
psychiatry, a new dynamic expertise, but
the position of the so-called mentally
ill remains unenviable,78; acts
conservatively, moulding the distressed
for roles as the disempowered 208; fails
to challenge the negative context in
which the 'mentally ill' live, 97; looks to
undermine the competence of survivors
152
psychosis, the meaning & experience of
treated dismissively xxviii; xxv–xxvi,
xxviii, xxxii, 19, 37, 59, 109, 114–121,
134–135, 220, 223
psychosurgery 155
psychotherapy 52
published letters to OpenMind magazine:
advocacy 65–66; coming through
[c.1983] 63–64; ECT: feared 65;
jabs & pills [c 1983] 63; professional
imperialism 64; regaining control 64;
the work ethic 65
punishment 203

quality of life 54

remoteness of psychiatric staff 47
Richmond Fellowship (RF) 47–48, 50, 61
Roberts, Andrew xxxi–xxxii, 224–226

Robinson, Georgina 111
Royal Dundee Liff Hospital 13–16

Sang, Bob 65–66
schizophrenia 19, 31, 51, 86
Schreber, Daniel Paul xxiii
seclusion xxvi, profound misgivings over
61, 137–139, 201
'Seclusion: The Bigger Picture' (2007)
201–202
self-advocacy 98–99, 193, 207; broader
view 102; broad sweep 102–103;
degrees of 100; levels of 99–100;
recipient view 101–102; user movement
100–101; 'Working Together For
Change' (1990) 98–103
self-control 103; loss of 40; resumption of
40
separation 32, 41
service user survivor groups 157–160
service user survivor movement 153–154,
207
sexual harassment in mental health services
112
shock therapies 155
sickness benefit forms 32
Silver Birch ward, Napsbury Hospital
173
social inclusion 159
social movements xxii
socio-political system 151
solitary confinement xix, xxix, 61, 113,
130, 137–139,140,151, 163, 166,
201–203
'Speaking for Ourselves' 206–209
spiritual crisis xxvi; with madness 59
'Spiritual crisis' (1993) 107–110
student-allocated observation 38
'Surviving Social Inclusion' (c 2000)
(Campbell) (Excerpted) 157–160
survivor-controlled initiative 152
survivor-led research 208
survivor movement xx, xxi–xxiv, xxvii,
xxxi, xxxiii,193–200, 206–210,
220–222
'The Survivor Movement in the 1980s'
(2006) 193–200
Survivors History Group 206
Survivors Poetry 194
Survivors Speak Out Edale Conference 59,
110, 206, 219
Szasz, Thomas 29

Moreover the diminished status we suffer while recovering from breakdown is not made right once we re-enter society. Discrimination affects us on major and minor levels, personal and public areas. Discrimination in employment is standard. There are many with psychiatric records who are forced to rinse their talents down the sink and take jobs far beneath their capabilities. I find it humiliating to have to lie in order to be in with a chance of work. To be advised to lie, to choose to do so and thereby admit a shame about my past which is not justified and which I in no way really feel has demeaned me more than any other single ~~f~~ event of my life outside hospital. I want a chance to be what I am and for that to be recognized as natural. Society is not only ignorant. It stuffs its ignorance down our throats as well.

My argument against the psychiatric system is not that it is uncaring. I have met individuals at all levels - nurse, social worker, psychiatrist - who were clearly caring people and have cared for me. But psychiatry must surely be more than custody and care. By approaching my situation in terms of illness, by regarding me primarily as a recipient of care and treatment, the system has consistently underestimated my capacity to change and ignored the potential it may contain to assist that change. My desire to win my own control of my breakdown process and thereby to gain independence and

For Product Safety Concerns and Information please contact our EU
representative GPSR@taylorandfrancis.com
Taylor & Francis Verlag GmbH, Kaufingerstraße 24, 80331 München, Germany

www.ingramcontent.com/pod-product-compliance
Lightning Source LLC
Chambersburg PA
CBHW050413280326
41932CB00013BA/1838

9 7 8 1 0 4 1 0 6 6 4 5 3